ATLAS OF THE HUMAN BODY

Frederic H. Martini, Ph.D.
University of Hawaii

Michael J. Timmons, M.S.
Moraine Valley Community College

Robert B. Tallitsch, Ph.D.
Augustana College

Ralph T. Hutchings
Biomedical Photographer

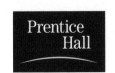

Pearson Education, Inc.,
Upper Saddle River, New Jersey 07458

Library of Congress Cataloging-in-Publication Data

Martini, Frederic.
    Atlas of the human body to accompany Human anatomy, 4th ed. / Frederic H. Martini,
Michael J. Timmons, Robert B. Tallitsch, with William C. Ober … [et al.].
        p. cm.
    ISBN 0-13-008906-0
    1. Human anatomy--Atlases.   I. Timmons, Michael J.   II. Tallitsch, Robert B.
    III. Martini, Frederic. Human body, 4th ed.   IV. Title.

QM23.2.M356 2003 Suppl.
611'.0022'3--dc21

                                            2002030721
                                            Rev.

Senior Editor: Halee Dinsey
Production Editor: Prepare, Inc.
Executive Managing Editor: Kathleen Schiaparelli
Assistant Managing Editor: Beth Sweeten
AV Editor: Adam Velthaus
Art Studio: Patty Gutierrez
Cover Designer: Alamini Design
Cover Illustration: Vincent Perez
Manufacturing Manager: Trudy Pisciotti
Manufacturing Buyer: Alan Fischer
Vice President of Production and Manufacturing: David W. Riccardi

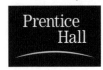

© 2003 Pearson Education, Inc.
Pearson Education, Inc.
Upper Saddle River, New Jersey 07458

Printed in the United States of America
10 9 8 7 6 5 4 3 2

ISBN 0-13-008906-0

Pearson Education LTD., *London*
Pearson Education Australia PTY, Limited, *Sydney*
Pearson Education Singapore, Pte. Ltd
Pearson Education North Asia Ltd, *Hong Kong*
Pearson Education Canada, Ltd., *Toronto*
Pearson Educación de Mexico, *S.A. de C.V.*
Pearson Education—Japan, *Tokyo*

CONTENTS

SCANS   **S-1**

1a MRI scan of the brain, horizontal section   S-2
1b MRI scan of the brain, horizontal section   S-2
1c MRI scan of the brain, horizontal section   S-2
1d MRI scan of the brain, parasagittal section   S-2
1e MRI scan of the brain, midsagittal section   S-2
2a MRI scan of the brain, coronal section   S-3
2b MRI scan of the brain, coronal section   S-3
2c MRI scan of the brain, coronal section   S-3
2d MRI scan of the brain, coronal section   S-3
3a MRI scan of the cervical vertebrae,
    anterior-posterior view   S-4
3b MRI scan of the vertebral column,
    sagittal section   S-4
4   MRI scan of the pelvis and hip joint,
    frontal section   S-4
5a MRI scan of the knee joint,
    horizontal section   S-5
5b MRI scan of the knee joint,
    horizontal section   S-5
6a MRI scan of the knee joint,
    parasagittal section   S-5
6b MRI scan of the knee joint,
    parasagittal section   S-5
7a MRI scan of the knee joint, frontal section   S-6
7b MRI scan of the knee joint, frontal section   S-6
8a MRI scan of the ankle joint,
    parasagittal section   S-6
8b MRI scan of the ankle joint,
    frontal section   S-6
9a MRI scan of the trunk, horizontal section   S-7
9b MRI scan of the trunk, horizontal section   S-7
9c MRI scan of the trunk, horizontal section   S-7
9d MRI scan of the trunk, horizontal section   S-8
9e MRI scan of the trunk, horizontal section   S-8
9f MRI scan of the trunk, horizontal section   S-8
9g CT scan of the trunk, horizontal section   S-9
9h CT scan of the trunk, horizontal section   S-9
9i CT scan of the trunk, horizontal section   S-9
10a 3-dimensional scan showing a fracture
    of the body of a lumbar vertebra   S-10
10b 3-dimensional scan of the elbow joint,
    superior view   S-10
10c Lymphangiogram of thorax,
    posterior view   S-10
10d 3-dimensional scan showing the use
    of a stent within the abdominal aorta
    and common iliac arteries   S-10

BONE IMAGES   **B-1**

1.1   The axial skeleton, anterior view   B-2
1.2   The axial skeleton, posterior view   B-2
2.1   The skeleton, anterior view   B-3
2.2   The skeleton, posterior view   B-3
3.1   Painted skull, anterolateral view   B-4
3.2   Painted skull, medial view   B-4
3.3   Painted skull, lateral view   B-5
3.4   The orbital bones   B-5
4.1   Fetal skull, anterior view   B-6
4.2a Infant skull, anterosuperior view   B-6

4.2b Infant skull, posterior view   B-6
5.1a Adult skull, posterior view   B-6
5.1b Adult skull, superior view   B-6
5.2   Adult skull, lateral view   B-7
5.3   Adult skull, anterior view   B-8
5.4   Adult skull, inferior view,
      mandible removed   B-9
5.5   Adult skull, horizontal section   B-10
5.6   Adult skull, sagittal section   B-11
6.1a Occipital bone, inferior (external) view   B-12
6.1b Occipital bone, superior (internal) view   B-12
6.2   Parietal bone, lateral view   B-13
6.3a Frontal bone, anterior view   B-13
6.3b Frontal bone, inferior view   B-13
6.3c Frontal bone, posterior (internal) view   B-14
6.4a Temporal bone, right temporal bone,
      lateral view   B-14
6.4b Temporal bone, right temporal bone,
      medial view   B-14
6.5a Sphenoid, superior surface   B-15
6.5b Sphenoid, anterior surface   B-15
6.6a Ethmoid, superior view   B-15
6.6b Ethmoid, posterior view   B-15
6.7   Cranial fossae, superior view   B-16
6.8a Right maxilla, lateral view   B-16
6.8b Right maxilla, medial view   B-16
6.9a Right palatine bone, medial view   B-17
6.9b Right palatine bone, lateral view   B-17
6.10a Mandible, lateral view   B-17
6.10b Mandible, medial view   B-17
6.11 Hyoid bone, anterior view   B-17
7.1   Vertebral column, lateral view   B-18
7.2a Cervical vertebrae, lateral view   B-18
7.2b Thoracic vertebrae, lateral view   B-18
7.2c Lumbar vertebrae, lateral view   B-19
7.3a Thoracic vertebra and rib, superior view   B-19
7.3b Rib, posterior and medial view   B-19
7.4   Thoracic cage, anterior view   B-20
8.1   Pectoral girdle and right upper limb,
      anterior view   B-21
8.2   Pelvic girdle and right lower limb,
      lateral view   B-21
8.3a Right clavicle, superior view   B-22
8.3b Right clavicle, inferior view   B-22
8.4   Right pectoral girdle, superior view   B-22
8.5a Right scapula, anterior view   B-23
8.5b Right scapula, lateral view   B-23
8.5c Right scapula, posterior view   B-23
8.6a Right humerus, anterior view   B-24
8.6b Right humerus, proximal, superior view   B-24
8.6c Right humerus, distal, inferior view   B-24
8.6d Right humerus, posterior view   B-25
8.7a Right radius and ulna, anterior view   B-25
8.7b Right radius and ulna, posterior view   B-25
8.8a Right elbow joint, posterior view   B-26
8.8b Right elbow joint, anterior view   B-26
8.8c Right ulna, proximal, lateral view   B-26
8.8d Right elbow joint, articular surfaces   B-26
8.9   Right wrist, anterior (palmar) view   B-27
8.10a Right hand, anterior (palmar) view   B-27
8.10b Right hand, posterior (dorsal) view   B-27

9.1a Pelvic girdle, lateral view   B-28
9.1b Pelvic girdle, medial view   B-29
9.2a Right femur, proximal, medial view   B-30
9.2b Right femur, proximal, lateral view   B-30
9.3a Right femur, superior view   B-30
9.3b Right femur, inferior view   B-30
9.4a Right tibia and fibula, anterior views   B-31
9.4b Right tibia, superior view   B-31
9.4c Right tibia and fibula, distal,
      inferior view   B-31
9.4d The tibia and fibula, posterior views   B-31
9.5a Right foot, superior (dorsal) view   B-32
9.5b Right foot, inferior (plantar) view   B-32
9.5c Right foot, lateral view   B-33
9.5d Right foot, medial view   B-33

CADAVER IMAGES   **C-1**

1.1   Superficial dissection of the face,
      lateral view   C-2
1.2   Deep dissection of the neck, lateral view   C-2
1.3   Surface anatomy of the anterior neck   C-3
1.4   Dissection of the anterior neck   C-3
1.5   Shoulder and neck, anterior view   C-3
2.1   The head in horizontal section   C-4
2.2   The head in sagittal section   C-5
3.1   Trunk, anterior view   C-6
3.2   Trunk, posterior view   C-7
4.1   The heart and lungs, anterior view   C-8
4.2a Right lung, medial view   C-8
4.2b Left lung, medial view   C-8
4.3a Painted segments of the right lung,
      anterior view   C-9
4.3b Painted segments of the left lung,
      anterior view   C-9
5.1   Abdominal wall, anterior view   C-9
5.2   Abdominal muscles   C-10
5.3a Abdominal dissection, superior portion,
      anterior view   C-10
5.3b Abdominal dissection, inferior portion,
      anterior view   C-11
5.3c Abdominal dissection,
      greater omentum reflected   C-11
5.3d Abdominal dissection, duodenal region   C-12
5.3e Appendix in situ   C-12
5.4a Liver and gallbladder, superior view   C-13
5.4b Liver and gallbladder, inferior view   C-13
5.4c Liver and gallbladder in situ   C-14
5.4d Corrosion cast of liver   C-14
5.5   Normal and abnormal colonoscope   C-15
5.6a Spleen, anterior view   C-15
5.6b Cast of splenic and pancreatic vessels   C-15
5.7a Superior mesenteric artery   C-16
5.7b Inferior mesenteric vessels   C-16
5.8a Abdominal cavity,
      horizontal section at T_{12} C-17
5.8b Abdominal cavity,
      horizontal section at L_1 C-18
5.9   The kidneys and associated structures   C-19
5.10a The inferior pelvis, superior view   C-20
5.10b Vessels of inferior pelvis, medial view   C-21

6.1	Right lower quadrant, male	C-21
6.2	Right hip, superficial dissection, posterior view	C-22
6.3	Right hip and thigh, anterior view	C-22
6.4a	Right foot, superficial dissection, lateral view	C-23
6.4b	Right foot, intrinsic muscles (superficial), plantar view	C-23
6.5a	Model of the right hand, posterior view	C-24
6.5b	Model of the elbow joint, longitudinal section	C-24
6.5c	Model of the knee joint, sagittal section	C-24

HISTOLOGY IMAGES   H-1

1.1	Simple columnar epithelium with goblet cells (LM×480)	H-2
1.2	Simple cuboidal and simple squamous epithelium (LM×240)	H-2
1.3	Stratified squamous epithelium (LM×240)	H-2
1.4	Stratified columnar epithelium (LM×480)	H-2
1.5	Pseudostratified columnar epithelium (LM×480)	H-2
1.6	Transitional epithelium (urinary bladder) (LM×480)	H-2
2.1	Pancreatic islets (islets of Langerhans) (LM×480)	H-3
2.2	Areolar connective tissue (mesenteric spread) (LM×480)	H-3
2.3	Dense irregular connective tissue (dermis of the skin) (LM×480)	H-3
2.4	Tendon (dense regular connective tissue) (LM×240)	H-3
2.5	Hyaline cartilage (trachea) (LM×240)	H-3
2.6	Elastic cartilage (auricle of the ear) (elastin stain) (LM×480)	H-3
3.1	Fibrocartilage (pubic symphysis) (LM×240)	H-4
3.2	Intramembranous (membrane) bone development (fetal pig) (LM×240)	H-4
3.3	Endochondral ossification at the epiphyseal cartilage (fetal metatarsal bone) (LM×48)	H-4
3.4	Bone spicule within the diaphysis of the developing bone (LM×240)	H-4
3.5	Compact bone (cross section), ground bone (LM×120)	H-4
3.6	Trabecular (cancellous) bone (LM×240)	H-4
4.1	Skeletal muscle (cross section) (LM×480)	H-5
4.2	Skeletal muscle (longitudinal section) (LM×480)	H-5
4.3	Cardiac muscle (LM×480)	H-5
4.4	Smooth muscle (longitudinal and cross sections) (LM×480)	H-5
4.5	Cerebellum (LM×120)	H-5
4.6	Purkinje cells of the cerebellum (silver stain) (LM×480)	H-5
5.1	Peripheral nerve (cross section) (LM×110)	H-6
5.2	Purkinje fibers within ventricle of human heart (LM×110)	H-6
5.3	Cross section of artery and vein (LM×110)	H-6
5.4	Capillaries within adipose tissue (LM×440)	H-6
5.5	Lung: transition from a terminal bronchiole to a respiratory bronchiole (LM×65)	H-6
5.6	Lung: alveolar duct (LM×65)	H-6
6.1	Lung: pulmonary alveoli (LM×220)	H-7
6.2	Aggregated lymphoid nodules (Peyer's patches) of ileum (LM×120)	H-7
6.3	Lymph node (LM×120)	H-7
6.4	Thymus of a child with Hassall's corpuscles (LM×120)	H-7
6.5	Atrophic thymus of an adult (LM×120)	H-7
6.6	Spleen (LM×120)	H-7
7.1	Kidney cortex: renal corpuscle, proximal and distal convoluted tubules (LM×500)	H-8
7.2	Thyroid gland (LM×50)	H-8
7.3	Endocrine pancreas: pancreatic islets (islets of Langerhans) (LM×200)	H-8
7.4	Testis (LM×50)	H-8
7.5	Primordial and primary follicles within the ovary (LM×50)	H-8
7.6	Graafian follicle within the ovary (LM×50)	H-8
8.1	Fundus of stomach (LM×50)	H-9
8.2	Ileum of small intestine (LM×50)	H-9
8.3	Colon (LM×50)	H-9
8.4	Appendix (LM×50)	H-9
8.5	Gallbladder (LM×50)	H-9
8.6	Liver (LM×50)	H-9

ILLUSTRATION CREDITS

Scans

1a-e, 2a-d, 3a-b, 4, 5a-b, 6a-b, 7a-b, 8a-b, 9a-f, 9g-i   Courtesy of Dr. Eugene C. Wasson, III, and staff of Maui Radiology Consultants, Maui Memorial Hospital

10a-b, d   Picker International

10c   Kathleen Welch, M.D.

Bones

1, 2, 3.1-3.3, 3.4, 4.1- 4.3, 5.1-5.5, 6.1-6.4b, 6.5a, 6.6-6.8a, 6.9a-6.18, 7.1-7.3, 7.5a-f, 8.1- 8.4, 8.6-8.19, 9.1-9.11   Ralph T. Hutchings

4.2   Michael J. Timmons

8.3   Bates/Custom Medical Stock Photo, Inc.

Cadavers

1.1, 1.2, 1.4, 1.5, 2.1, 2.2, 3.1, 3.2, 4.1, 4.2a-b, 4.3a-b, 5.1, 5.2, 5.2b, 5.3a-d, 5.4a-d, 5.5, 5.6a-b, 5.7a-b, 5.8a-b, 5.9, 5.10a-b, 6.1, 6.2, 6.3, 6.4a, 6.4b   Ralph T. Hutchings

6.6a, 8.12d, 6.5c   Patrick M. Timmons/Michael J. Timmons

1.3   University of Toronto

Histology

All histology images courtesy of Robert B. Tallitsch, Ph.D. with Ronald Guastaferri, B.A., M.A.M.S.

SCANS

FIGURE 1a   MRI SCAN OF THE BRAIN, HORIZONTAL SECTION S-2

FIGURE 1b   MRI SCAN OF THE BRAIN, HORIZONTAL SECTION S-2

FIGURE 1c   MRI SCAN OF THE BRAIN, HORIZONTAL SECTION S-2

FIGURE 1d   MRI SCAN OF THE BRAIN, PARASAGITTAL SECTION S-2

FIGURE 1e   MRI SCAN OF THE BRAIN, MIDSAGITTAL SECTION S-2

FIGURE 2a   MRI SCAN OF THE BRAIN, CORONAL SECTION S-3

FIGURE 2b   MRI SCAN OF THE BRAIN, CORONAL SECTION S-3

FIGURE 2c   MRI SCAN OF THE BRAIN, CORONAL SECTION S-3

FIGURE 2d   MRI SCAN OF THE BRAIN, CORONAL SECTION S-3

FIGURE 3a   MRI SCAN OF THE CERVICAL VERTEBRAE,
ANTERIOR–POSTERIOR VIEW S-4

FIGURE 3b   MRI SCAN OF THE VERTEBRAL COLUMN,
SAGITTAL SECTION S-4

FIGURE 4   MRI SCAN OF THE PELVIS AND HIP JOINT,
FRONTAL SECTION S-4

FIGURE 5a   MRI SCAN OF THE KNEE JOINT, HORIZONTAL SECTION . S-5

FIGURE 5b   MRI SCAN OF THE KNEE JOINT, HORIZONTAL SECTION . S-5

FIGURE 6a   MRI SCAN OF THE KNEE JOINT, PARASAGITTAL SECTION   S-5

FIGURE 6b   MRI SCAN OF THE KNEE JOINT, PARASAGITTAL SECTION   S-5

FIGURE 7a   MRI SCAN OF THE KNEE JOINT, FRONTAL SECTION S-6

FIGURE 7b   MRI SCAN OF THE KNEE JOINT, FRONTAL SECTION S-6

FIGURE 8a   MRI SCAN OF THE ANKLE JOINT, PARASAGITTAL SECTION   S-6

FIGURE 8b   MRI SCAN OF THE ANKLE JOINT, FRONTAL SECTION . . . S-6

FIGURE 9a   MRI SCAN OF THE TRUNK, HORIZONTAL SECTION S-7

FIGURE 9b   MRI SCAN OF THE TRUNK, HORIZONTAL SECTION S-7

FIGURE 9c   MRI SCAN OF THE TRUNK, HORIZONTAL SECTION S-7

FIGURE 9d   MRI SCAN OF THE TRUNK, HORIZONTAL SECTION S-8

FIGURE 9e   MRI SCAN OF THE TRUNK, HORIZONTAL SECTION S-8

FIGURE 9f   MRI SCAN OF THE TRUNK, HORIZONTAL SECTION S-8

FIGURE 9g   CT SCAN OF THE TRUNK, HORIZONTAL SECTION S-9

FIGURE 9h   CT SCAN OF THE TRUNK, HORIZONTAL SECTION S-9

FIGURE 9i   CT SCAN OF THE TRUNK, HORIZONTAL SECTION S-9

FIGURE 10a   3-DIMENSIONAL SCAN SHOWING A FRACTURE
OF THE BODY OF A LUMBAR VERTEBRA S-10

FIGURE 10b   3-DIMENSIONAL SCAN OF THE ELBOW JOINT,
SUPERIOR VIEW S-10

FIGURE 10c   LYMPHANGIOGRAM OF THORAX, POSTERIOR VIEW S-10

FIGURE 10d   3-DIMENSIONAL SCAN SHOWING THE USE
OF A STENT WITHIN THE ABDOMINAL AORTA
AND COMMON ILIAC ARTERIES S-10

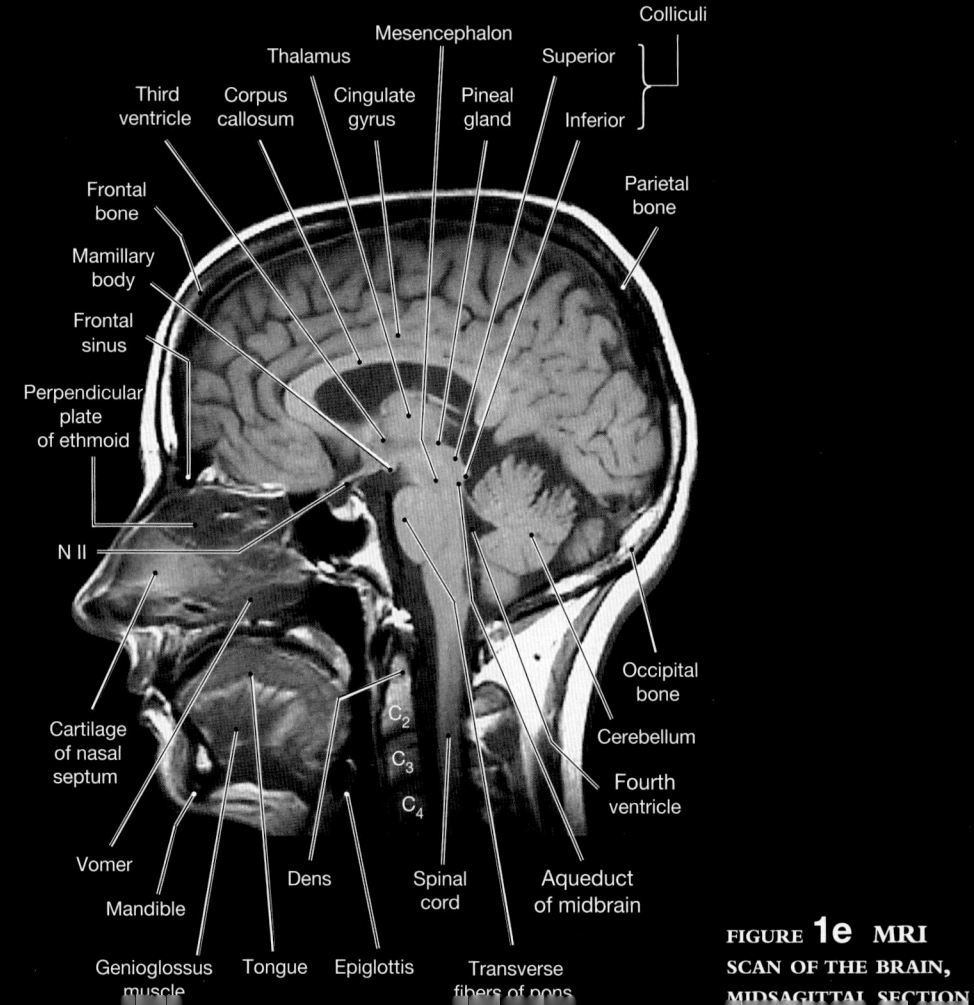

Septum pellucidum
Longitudinal fissure
Lateral ventricles

FIGURE 1a MRI SCAN OF THE BRAIN, HORIZONTAL SECTION

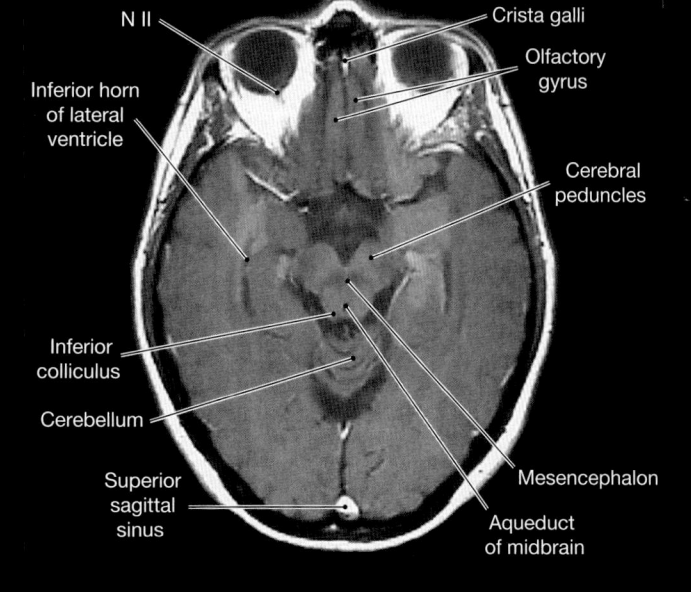

N II
Crista galli
Olfactory gyrus
Inferior horn of lateral ventricle
Cerebral peduncles
Inferior colliculus
Cerebellum
Superior sagittal sinus
Mesencephalon
Aqueduct of midbrain

FIGURE 1b MRI SCAN OF THE BRAIN, HORIZONTAL SECTION

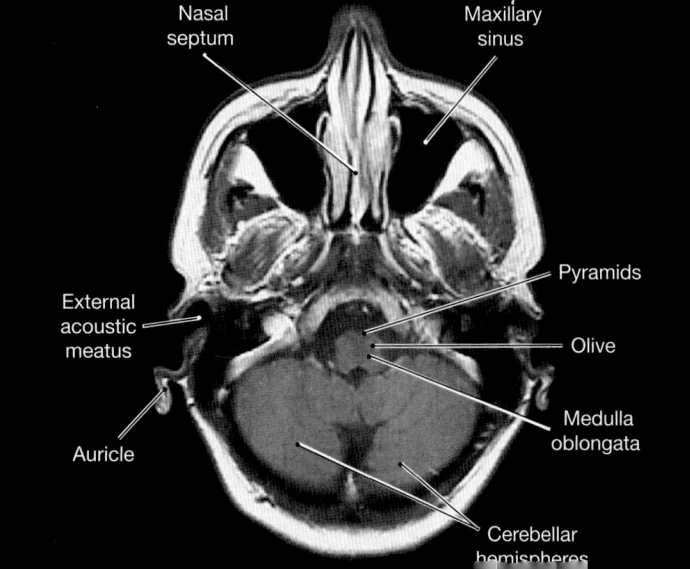

Nasal septum
Maxillary sinus
External acoustic meatus
Pyramids
Olive
Medulla oblongata
Auricle
Cerebellar hemispheres

FIGURE 1c MRI SCAN OF THE BRAIN, HORIZONTAL SECTION

Lateral sulcus
Parietal lobe (left)
Posterior horn of lateral ventricle
Frontal lobe (left)
Skull
Occipital lobe (left)
Posterior cavity of left eye
Pupil
Extra-ocular muscles
Maxillary sinus
Cerebellum
Splenius capitis muscle
Trapezius muscle

FIGURE 1d MRI SCAN OF THE BRAIN, PARASAGITTAL SECTION

Third ventricle
Corpus callosum
Thalamus
Mesencephalon
Cingulate gyrus
Pineal gland
Superior
Colliculi
Inferior
Frontal bone
Mamillary body
Frontal sinus
Parietal bone
Perpendicular plate of ethmoid
N II
Cartilage of nasal septum
C₂
C₃
C₄
Occipital bone
Cerebellum
Fourth ventricle
Vomer
Dens
Spinal cord
Aqueduct of midbrain
Mandible
Genioglossus muscle
Tongue
Epiglottis
Transverse fibers of pons

FIGURE 1e MRI SCAN OF THE BRAIN, MIDSAGITTAL SECTION

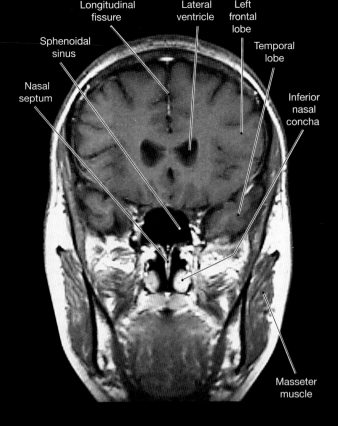

Longitudinal fissure
Lateral ventricle
Left frontal lobe
Temporal lobe
Sphenoidal sinus
Inferior nasal concha
Nasal septum
Masseter muscle

FIGURE **2a** MRI SCAN OF THE BRAIN, CORONAL SECTION

Septum pellucidum
Corpus callosum
Superior sagittal sinus
Third ventricle
Interventricular foramen
Thalamus
Insula
Lateral sulcus
Temporal lobe

FIGURE **2b** MRI SCAN OF THE BRAIN, CORONAL SECTION

FIGURE **2c** MRI SCAN OF THE BRAIN, CORONAL SECTION

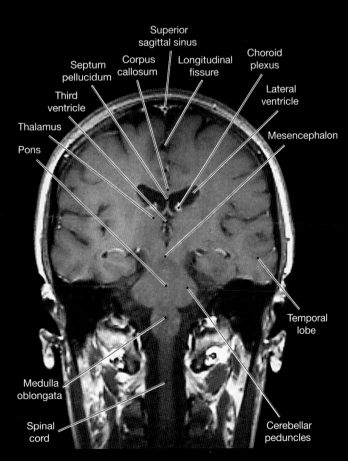

Superior sagittal sinus
Septum pellucidum
Corpus callosum
Longitudinal fissure
Choroid plexus
Third ventricle
Lateral ventricle
Thalamus
Mesencephalon
Pons
Temporal lobe
Medulla oblongata
Spinal cord
Cerebellar peduncles

FIGURE **2d** MRI SCAN OF THE BRAIN, CORONAL SECTION

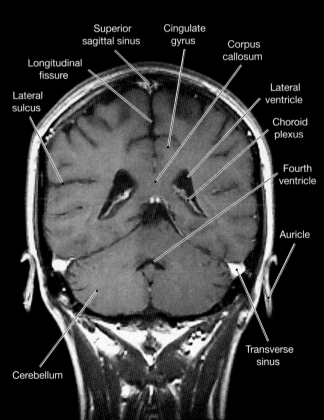

Superior sagittal sinus
Cingulate gyrus
Corpus callosum
Longitudinal fissure
Lateral sulcus
Lateral ventricle
Choroid plexus
Fourth ventricle
Auricle
Cerebellum
Transverse sinus

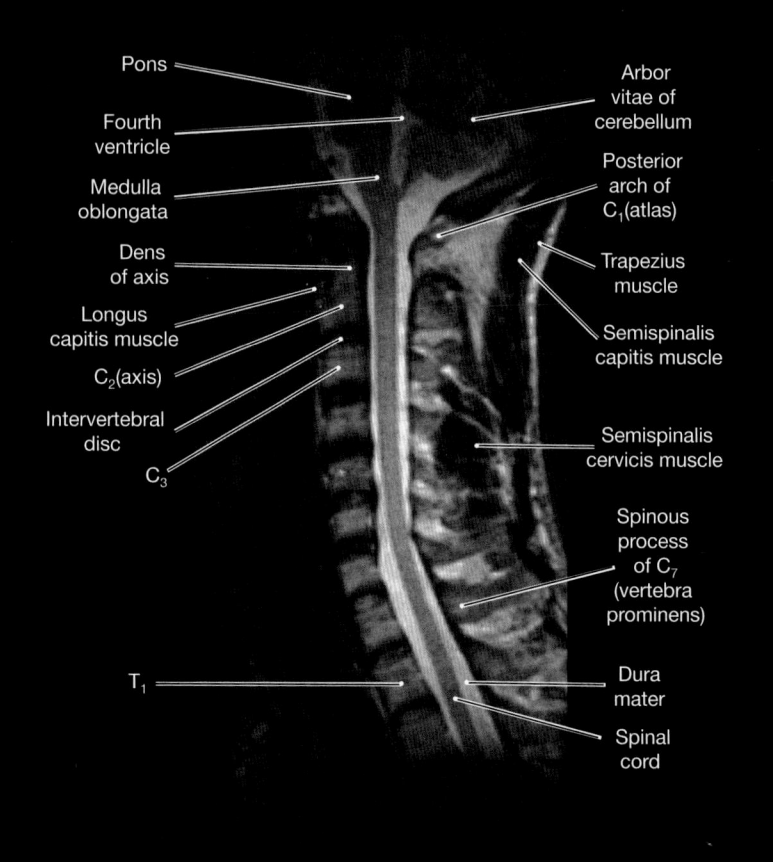

Pons

Fourth ventricle

Medulla oblongata

Dens of axis

Longus capitis muscle

C_2(axis)

Intervertebral disc

C_3

T_1

Arbor vitae of cerebellum

Posterior arch of C_1(atlas)

Trapezius muscle

Semispinalis capitis muscle

Semispinalis cervicis muscle

Spinous process of C_7 (vertebra prominens)

Dura mater

Spinal cord

FIGURE 3a MRI SCAN OF THE CERVICAL VERTEBRAE, ANTERIOR– POSTERIOR VIEW

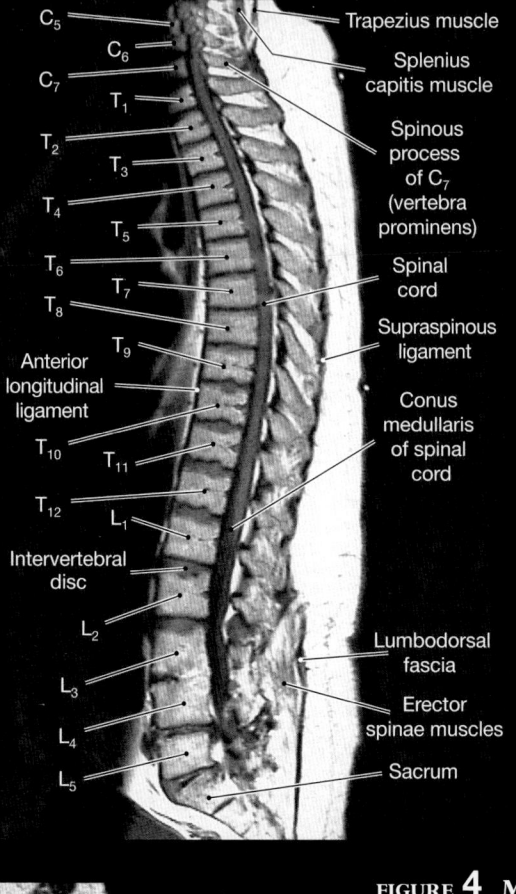

C_5
C_6
C_7
T_1
T_2
T_3
T_4
T_5
T_6
T_7
T_8
T_9

Anterior longitudinal ligament

T_{10}
T_{11}
T_{12}
L_1

Intervertebral disc

L_2
L_3
L_4
L_5

Trapezius muscle

Splenius capitis muscle

Spinous process of C_7 (vertebra prominens)

Spinal cord

Supraspinous ligament

Conus medullaris of spinal cord

Lumbodorsal fascia

Erector spinae muscles

Sacrum

FIGURE 3b MRI SCAN OF THE VERTEBRAL COLUMN, SAGITTAL SECTION

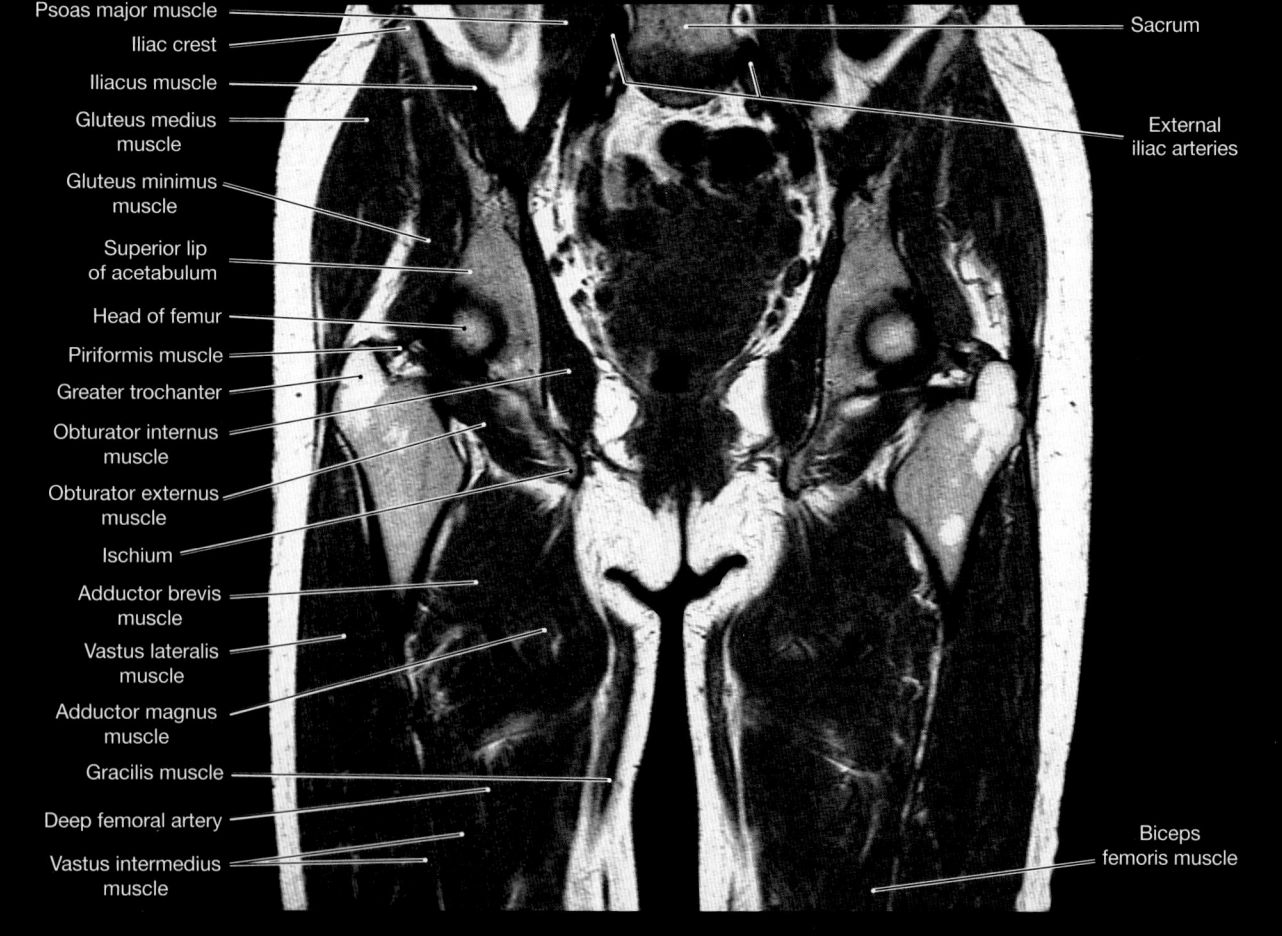

Psoas major muscle

Iliac crest

Iliacus muscle

Gluteus medius muscle

Gluteus minimus muscle

Superior lip of acetabulum

Head of femur

Piriformis muscle

Greater trochanter

Obturator internus muscle

Obturator externus muscle

Ischium

Adductor brevis muscle

Vastus lateralis muscle

Adductor magnus muscle

Gracilis muscle

Deep femoral artery

Vastus intermedius muscle

Sacrum

External iliac arteries

Biceps femoris muscle

FIGURE 4 MRI SCAN OF THE PELVIS AND HIP JOINT, FRONTAL SECTION

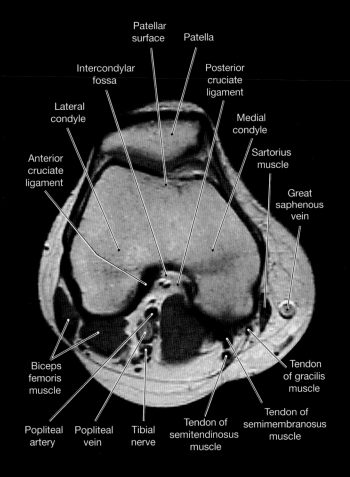

Patellar surface
Patella
Patellar surface
Intercondylar fossa
Posterior cruciate ligament
Lateral condyle
Medial condyle
Anterior cruciate ligament
Sartorius muscle
Great saphenous vein
Biceps femoris muscle
Tendon of gracilis muscle
Popliteal artery
Popliteal vein
Tibial nerve
Tendon of semitendinosus muscle
Tendon of semimembranosus muscle

FIGURE 5a MRI SCAN OF THE KNEE JOINT, HORIZONTAL SECTION

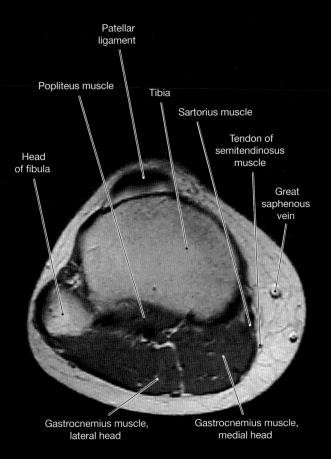

Patellar ligament
Popliteus muscle
Tibia
Sartorius muscle
Tendon of semitendinosus muscle
Head of fibula
Great saphenous vein
Gastrocnemius muscle, lateral head
Gastrocnemius muscle, medial head

FIGURE 5b MRI SCAN OF THE KNEE JOINT, HORIZONTAL SECTION

FIGURE 6a MRI SCAN OF THE KNEE JOINT, PARASAGITTAL SECTION

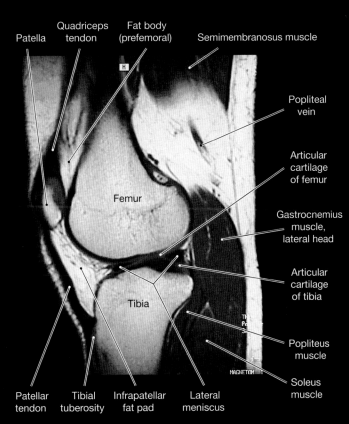

Patella
Quadriceps tendon
Fat body (prefemoral)
Semimembranosus muscle
Popliteal vein
Articular cartilage of femur
Femur
Gastrocnemius muscle, lateral head
Articular cartilage of tibia
Tibia
Popliteus muscle
Patellar tendon
Tibial tuberosity
Infrapatellar fat pad
Lateral meniscus
Soleus muscle

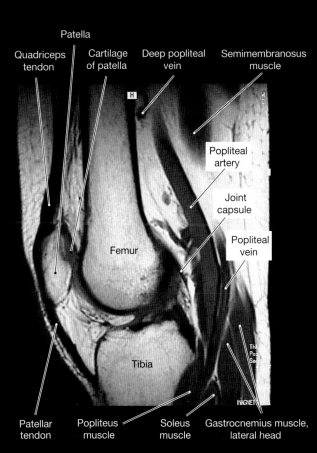

Patella
Quadriceps tendon
Cartilage of patella
Deep popliteal vein
Semimembranosus muscle
Popliteal artery
Joint capsule
Popliteal vein
Femur
Tibia
Patellar tendon
Popliteus muscle
Soleus muscle
Gastrocnemius muscle, lateral head

FIGURE 6b MRI SCAN OF THE KNEE JOINT, PARASAGITTAL SECTION

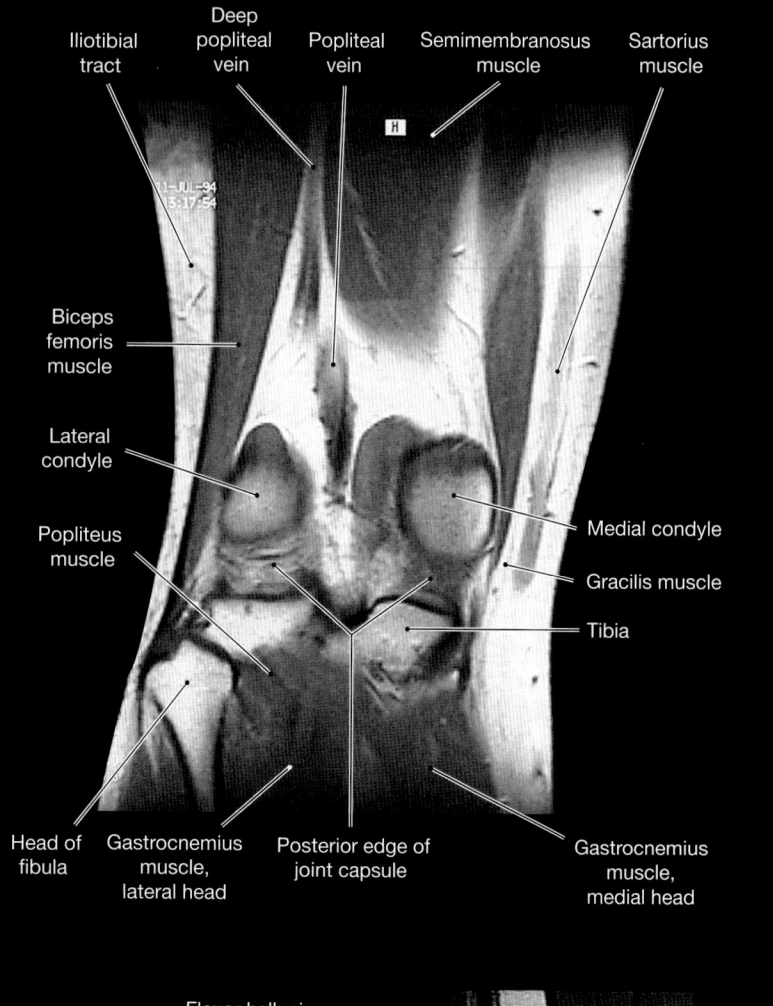

Iliotibial tract
Deep popliteal vein
Popliteal vein
Semimembranosus muscle
Sartorius muscle

Biceps femoris muscle

Lateral condyle

Popliteus muscle

Medial condyle

Gracilis muscle

Tibia

Head of fibula
Gastrocnemius muscle, lateral head
Posterior edge of joint capsule
Gastrocnemius muscle, medial head

FIGURE **7a** MRI SCAN OF THE KNEE JOINT, FRONTAL SECTION

Anterior cruciate ligament
Biceps femoris muscle
Popliteal vein
Intercondylar fossa
Vastus medialis muscle
Posterior cruciate ligament

Lateral condyle of femur

Fibular collateral ligament

Lateral meniscus

Medial condyle of femur

Medial meniscus

Tibia

Tibial collateral ligament

Tubercles of intercondylar eminence of tibia
Epiphyseal line
Gastrocnemius muscle, medial head
Great saphenous vein

FIGURE **7b** MRI SCAN OF THE KNEE JOINT, FRONTAL SECTION

FIGURE **8a** MRI SCAN OF THE ANKLE JOINT, PARASAGITTAL SECTION

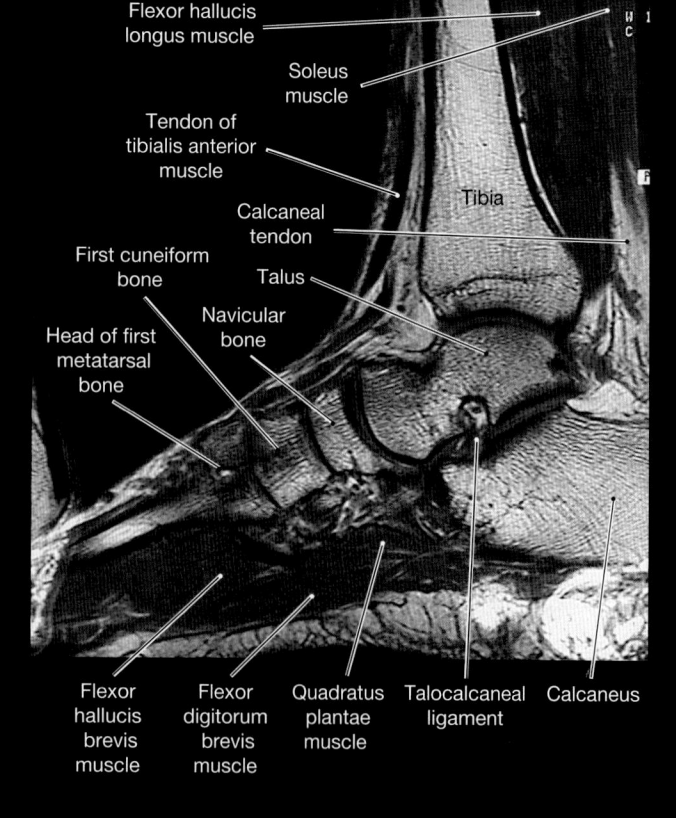

Flexor hallucis longus muscle
Soleus muscle
Tendon of tibialis anterior muscle
Calcaneal tendon
Tibia
First cuneiform bone
Talus
Navicular bone
Head of first metatarsal bone

Flexor hallucis brevis muscle
Flexor digitorum brevis muscle
Quadratus plantae muscle
Talocalcaneal ligament
Calcaneus

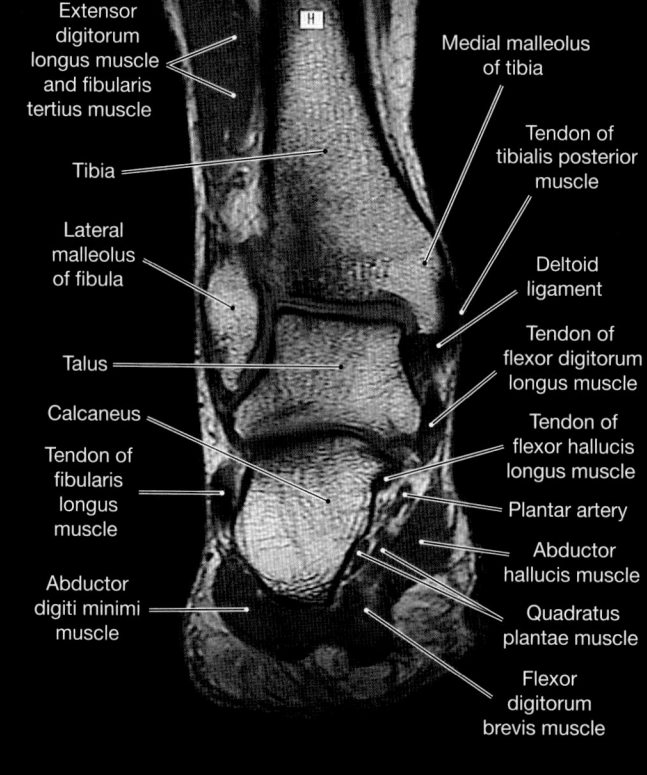

Extensor digitorum longus muscle and fibularis tertius muscle
Medial malleolus of tibia

Tibia

Tendon of tibialis posterior muscle

Lateral malleolus of fibula

Deltoid ligament

Talus

Tendon of flexor digitorum longus muscle

Calcaneus

Tendon of flexor hallucis longus muscle

Tendon of fibularis longus muscle

Plantar artery

Abductor hallucis muscle

Abductor digiti minimi muscle

Quadratus plantae muscle

Flexor digitorum brevis muscle

FIGURE **8b** MRI SCAN OF THE ANKLE JOINT, FRONTAL SECTION

FIGURE **9a** MRI
SCAN OF THE TRUNK,
HORIZONTAL SECTION

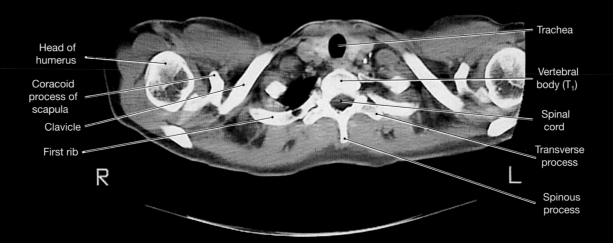

Head of humerus

Coracoid process of scapula

Clavicle

First rib

R

Trachea

Vertebral body (T$_1$)

Spinal cord

Transverse process

Spinous process

L

FIGURE **9b** MRI
SCAN OF THE TRUNK,
HORIZONTAL SECTION

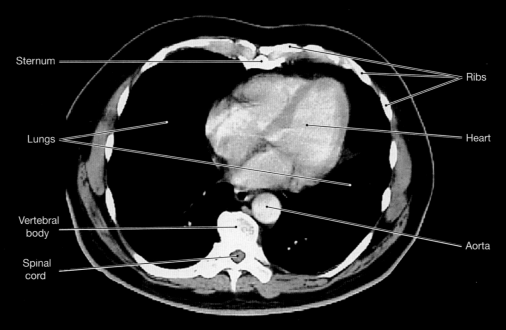

Sternum

Lungs

Vertebral body

Spinal cord

Ribs

Heart

Aorta

FIGURE **9c** MRI
SCAN OF THE TRUNK,
HORIZONTAL SECTION

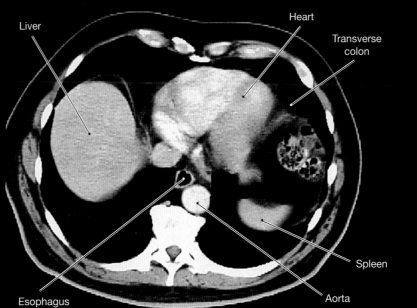

Liver

Heart

Transverse colon

Spleen

Esophagus

Aorta

FIGURE **9d** MRI
SCAN OF THE TRUNK,
HORIZONTAL SECTION

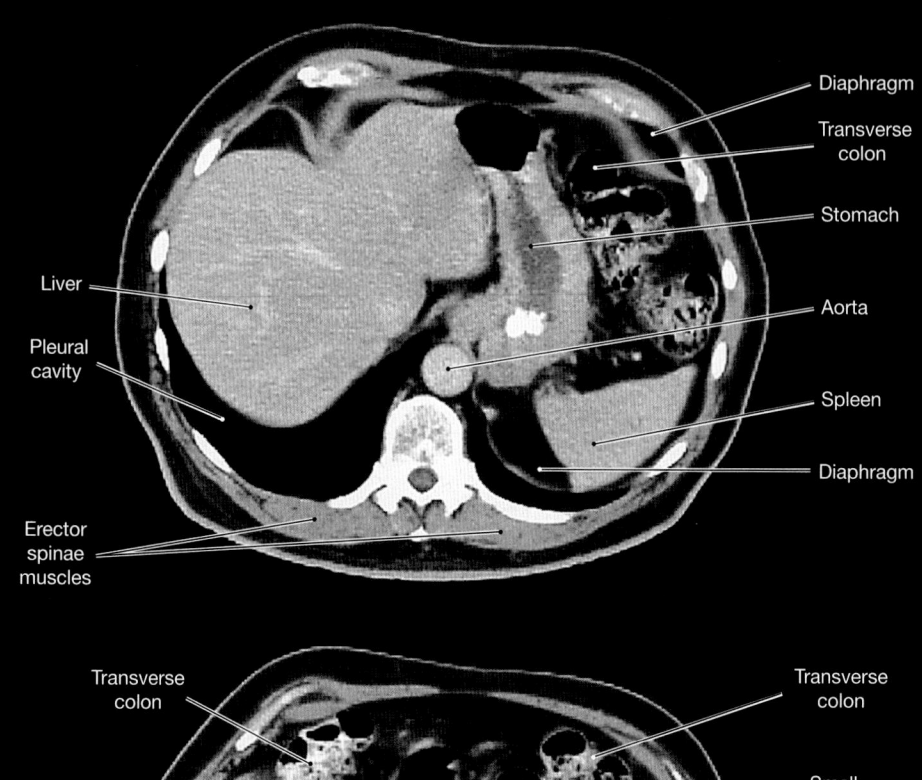

Diaphragm

Transverse
colon

Stomach

Liver

Aorta

Pleural
cavity

Spleen

Diaphragm

Erector
spinae
muscles

FIGURE **9e** MRI
SCAN OF THE TRUNK,
HORIZONTAL SECTION

Transverse
colon

Transverse
colon

Small
intestine

Aorta

Liver

Right
kidney

Spleen

Diaghragm

Left
kidney

FIGURE **9f** MRI SCAN
OF THE TRUNK,
HORIZONTAL SECTION

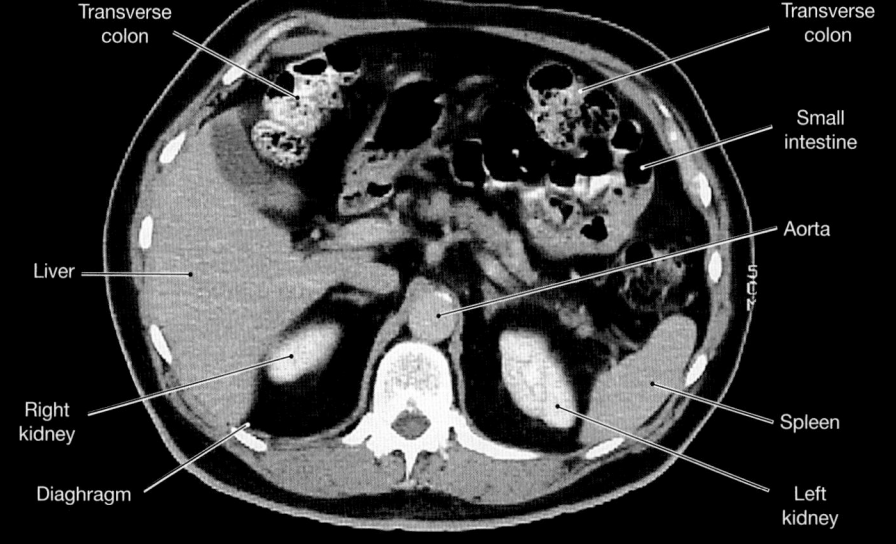

Transverse
colon

Superior
mesenteric
vein

Small
intestine

Colon

Superior
mesenteric
artery

Liver

Renal
vein

Pancreas

Aorta

Inferior
vena cava

Renal
artery

Renal
pelvis

Right
kidney

Left
kidney

Erector
spinae
muscles

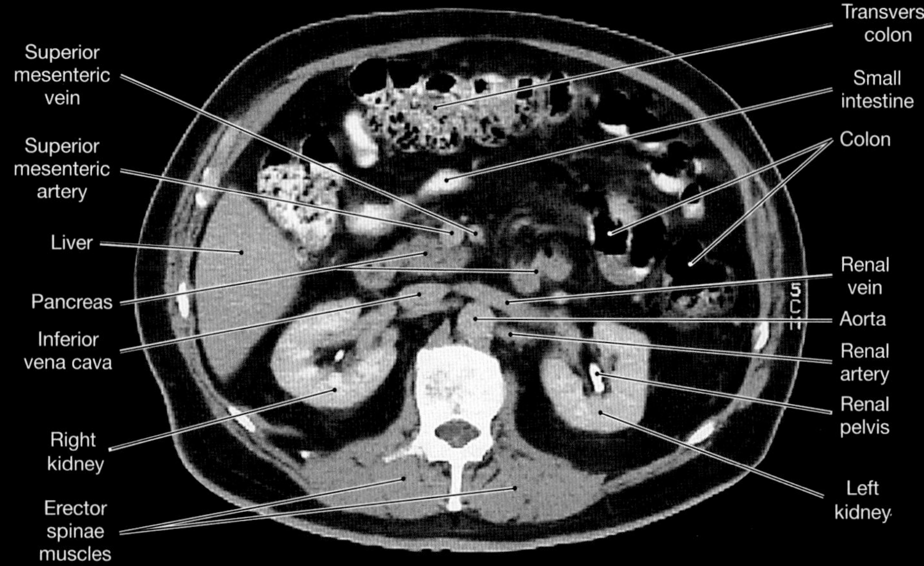

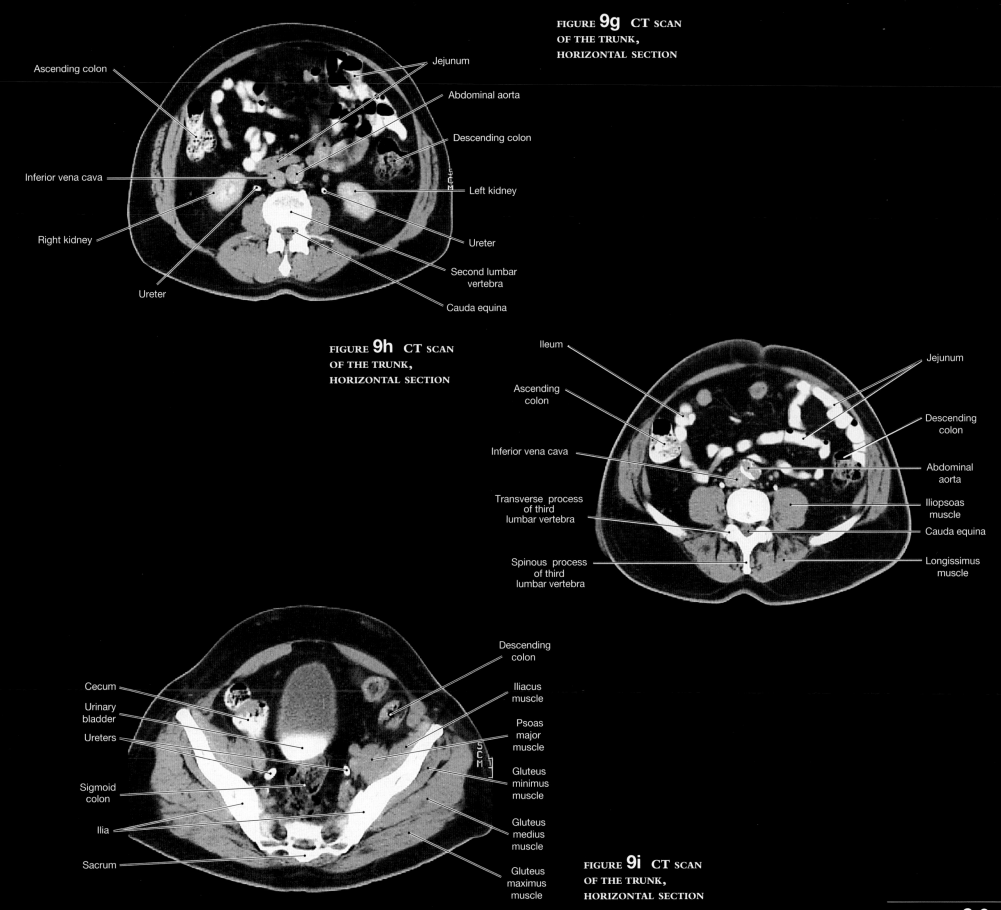

Ascending colon

Jejunum

Abdominal aorta

Descending colon

Inferior vena cava

Left kidney

Right kidney

Ureter

Ureter

Second lumbar vertebra

Cauda equina

FIGURE **9h** CT SCAN OF THE TRUNK, HORIZONTAL SECTION

Ileum

Jejunum

Ascending colon

Descending colon

Inferior vena cava

Abdominal aorta

Transverse process of third lumbar vertebra

Iliopsoas muscle

Cauda equina

Spinous process of third lumbar vertebra

Longissimus muscle

Descending colon

Cecum

Iliacus muscle

Urinary bladder

Psoas major muscle

Ureters

Gluteus minimus muscle

Sigmoid colon

Ilia

Gluteus medius muscle

Sacrum

Gluteus maximus muscle

FIGURE **9i** CT SCAN OF THE TRUNK, HORIZONTAL SECTION

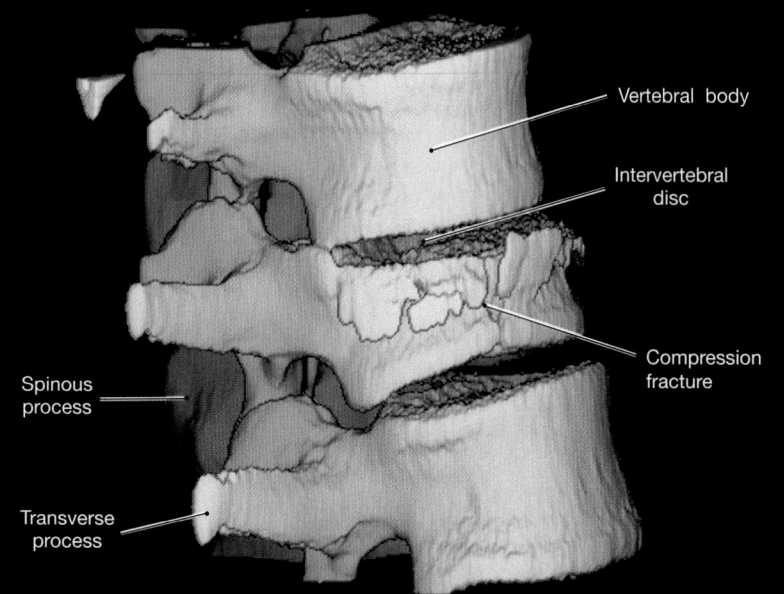

FIGURE 10a
3-DIMENSIONAL SCAN SHOWING FRACTURE OF THE BODY OF A LUMBAR VERTEBRA

Vertebral body

Intervertebral disc

Compression fracture

Spinous process

Transverse process

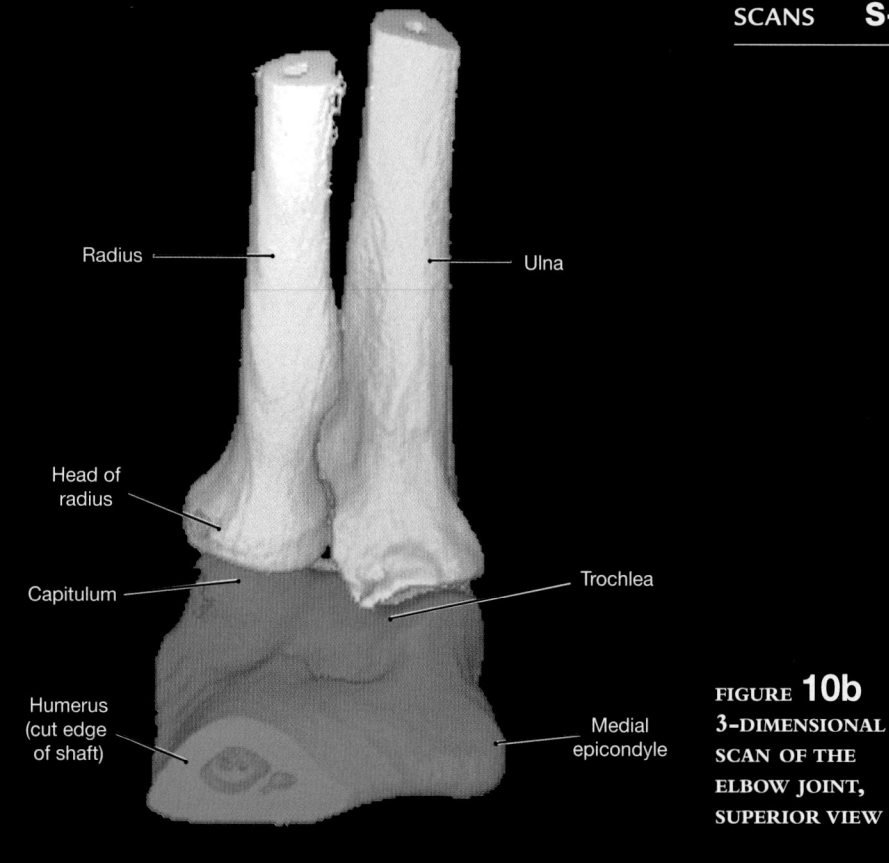

Radius

Ulna

Head of radius

Capitulum

Trochlea

Humerus (cut edge of shaft)

Medial epicondyle

FIGURE 10b
3-DIMENSIONAL SCAN OF THE ELBOW JOINT, SUPERIOR VIEW

FIGURE 10c
LYMPHANGIO-GRAM OF THORAX, POSTERIOR VIEW

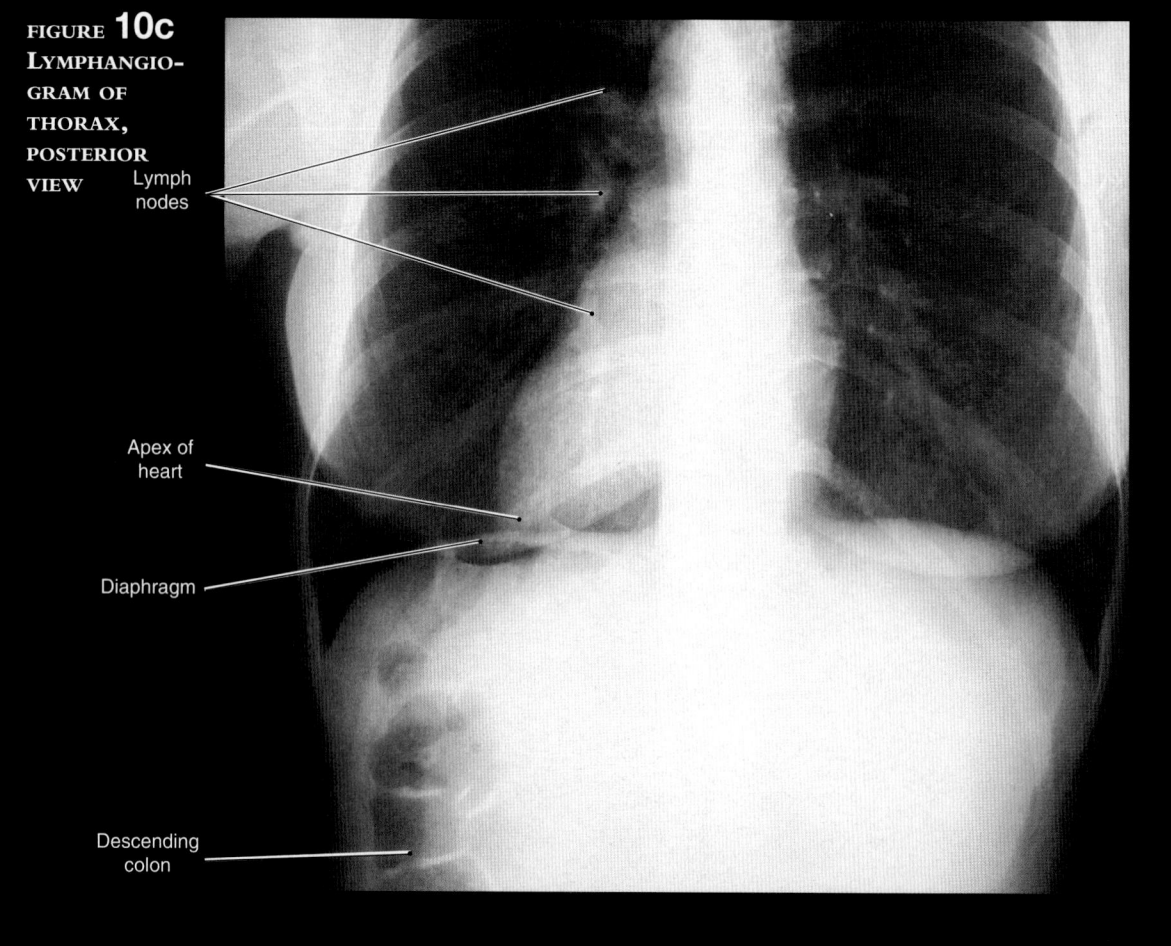

Lymph nodes

Apex of heart

Diaphragm

Descending colon

FIGURE 10d
3-DIMENSIONAL SCAN SHOWING THE USE OF A STENT WITHIN THE ABDOMINAL AORTA AND COMMON ILIAC ARTERIES

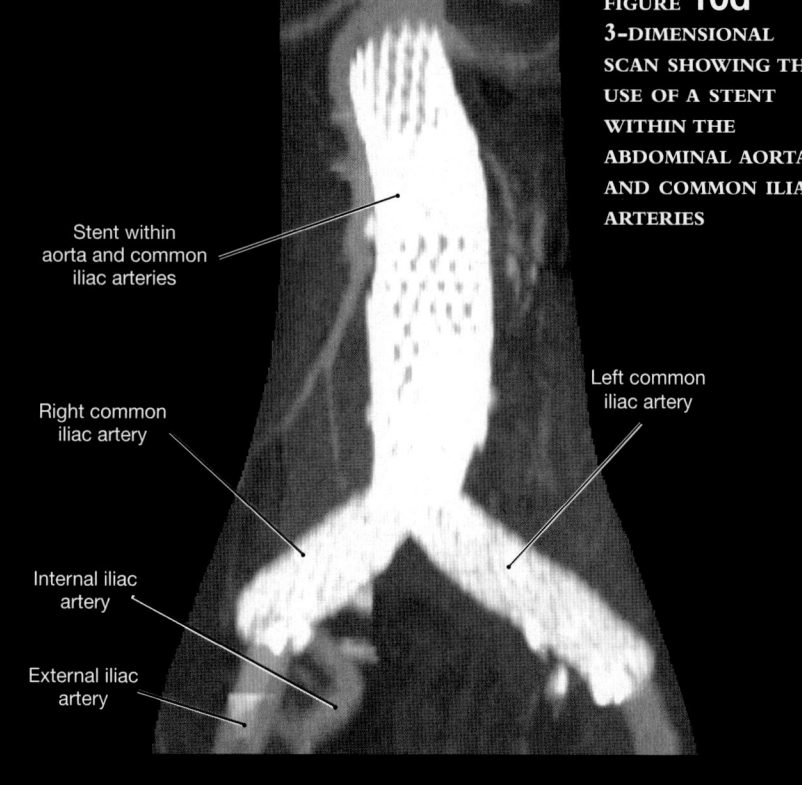

Stent within aorta and common iliac arteries

Left common iliac artery

Right common iliac artery

Internal iliac artery

External iliac artery

BONE IMAGES

FIGURE 1.1 THE AXIAL SKELETON, ANTERIOR VIEW B-2
FIGURE 1.2 THE AXIAL SKELETON, POSTERIOR VIEW B-2
FIGURE 2.1 THE SKELETON, ANTERIOR VIEW B-3
FIGURE 2.2 THE SKELETON, POSTERIOR VIEW B-3
FIGURE 3.1 PAINTED SKULL, ANTEROLATERAL VIEW B-4
FIGURE 3.2 PAINTED SKULL, MEDIAL VIEW B-4
FIGURE 3.3 PAINTED SKULL, LATERAL VIEW B-5
FIGURE 3.4 THE ORBITAL BONES B-5
FIGURE 4.1 FETAL SKULL, ANTERIOR VIEW B-6
FIGURE 4.2a INFANT SKULL, ANTEROSUPERIOR VIEW B-6
FIGURE 4.2b INFANT SKULL, POSTERIOR VIEW B-6
FIGURE 5.1a ADULT SKULL, POSTERIOR VIEW B-6
FIGURE 5.1b ADULT SKULL, SUPERIOR VIEW B-6
FIGURE 5.2 ADULT SKULL, LATERAL VIEW B-7
FIGURE 5.3 ADULT SKULL, ANTERIOR VIEW B-8
FIGURE 5.4 ADULT SKULL, INFERIOR VIEW, MANDIBLE REMOVED B-9
FIGURE 5.5 ADULT SKULL, HORIZONTAL SECTION B-10
FIGURE 5.6 ADULT SKULL, SAGITTAL SECTION B-11
FIGURE 6.1a OCCIPITAL BONE, INFERIOR (EXTERNAL) VIEW B-12
FIGURE 6.1b OCCIPITAL BONE, SUPERIOR (INTERNAL) VIEW B-12
FIGURE 6.2 PARIETAL BONE, LATERAL VIEW B-13
FIGURE 6.3a FRONTAL BONE, ANTERIOR VIEW B-13
FIGURE 6.3b FRONTAL BONE, INFERIOR VIEW B-13
FIGURE 6.3c FRONTAL BONE, POSTERIOR (INTERNAL) VIEW B-14
FIGURE 6.4a TEMPORAL BONE, RIGHT TEMPORAL BONE, LATERAL VIEW . B-14
FIGURE 6.4b TEMPORAL BONE, RIGHT TEMPORAL BONE, MEDIAL VIEW . . B-14
FIGURE 6.5a SPHENOID, SUPERIOR SURFACE B-15
FIGURE 6.5b SPHENOID, ANTERIOR SURFACE B-15
FIGURE 6.6a ETHMOID, SUPERIOR VIEW B-15
FIGURE 6.6b ETHMOID, POSTERIOR VIEW B-15
FIGURE 6.7 CRANIAL FOSSAE, SUPERIOR VIEW B-16
FIGURE 6.8a RIGHT MAXILLA, LATERAL VIEW B-16
FIGURE 6.8b RIGHT MAXILLA, MEDIAL VIEW B-16
FIGURE 6.9a RIGHT PALATINE BONE, MEDIAL VIEW B-17
FIGURE 6.9b RIGHT PALATINE BONE, LATERAL VIEW B-17
FIGURE 6.10a MANDIBLE, LATERAL VIEW B-17
FIGURE 6.10b MANDIBLE, MEDIAL VIEW B-17
FIGURE 6.11 HYOID BONE, ANTERIOR VIEW B-17
FIGURE 7.1 VERTEBRAL COLUMN, LATERAL VIEW B-18

FIGURE 7.2b THORACIC VERTEBRAE, LATERAL VIEW B-18
FIGURE 7.2c LUMBAR VERTEBRAE, LATERAL VIEW B-19
FIGURE 7.3a THORACIC VERTEBRA AND RIB, SUPERIOR VIEW B-19
FIGURE 7.3b RIB, POSTERIOR AND MEDIAL VIEW B-19
FIGURE 7.4 THORACIC CAGE, ANTERIOR VIEW B-20
FIGURE 8.1 PECTORAL GIRDLE AND RIGHT UPPER LIMB, ANTERIOR VIEW . B-21
FIGURE 8.2 PELVIC GIRDLE AND RIGHT LOWER LIMB, LATERAL VIEW . . B-21
FIGURE 8.3a RIGHT CLAVICLE, SUPERIOR VIEW B-22
FIGURE 8.3b RIGHT CLAVICLE, INFERIOR VIEW B-22
FIGURE 8.4 RIGHT PECTORAL GIRDLE, SUPERIOR VIEW B-22
FIGURE 8.5a RIGHT SCAPULA, ANTERIOR VIEW B-23
FIGURE 8.5b RIGHT SCAPULA, LATERAL VIEW B-23
FIGURE 8.5c RIGHT SCAPULA, POSTERIOR VIEW B-23
FIGURE 8.6a RIGHT HUMERUS, ANTERIOR VIEW B-24
FIGURE 8.6b RIGHT HUMERUS, PROXIMAL, SUPERIOR VIEW B-24
FIGURE 8.6c RIGHT HUMERUS, DISTAL, INFERIOR VIEW B-24
FIGURE 8.6d RIGHT HUMERUS, POSTERIOR VIEW B-25
FIGURE 8.7a RIGHT RADIUS AND ULNA, ANTERIOR VIEW B-25
FIGURE 8.7b RIGHT RADIUS AND ULNA, POSTERIOR VIEW B-25
FIGURE 8.8a RIGHT ELBOW JOINT, POSTERIOR VIEW B-26
FIGURE 8.8b RIGHT ELBOW JOINT, ANTERIOR VIEW B-26
FIGURE 8.8c RIGHT ULNA, PROXIMAL, LATERAL VIEW B-26
FIGURE 8.8d RIGHT ELBOW JOINT, ARTICULAR SURFACES B-26
FIGURE 8.9 RIGHT WRIST, ANTERIOR (PALMAR) VIEW B-27
FIGURE 8.10a RIGHT HAND, ANTERIOR (PALMAR) VIEW B-27
FIGURE 8.10b RIGHT HAND, POSTERIOR (DORSAL) VIEW B-27
FIGURE 9.1a PELVIC GIRDLE, LATERAL VIEW B-28
FIGURE 9.1b PELVIC GIRDLE, MEDIAL VIEW B-29
FIGURE 9.2a RIGHT FEMUR, PROXIMAL, MEDIAL VIEW B-30
FIGURE 9.2b RIGHT FEMUR, PROXIMAL, LATERAL VIEW B-30
FIGURE 9.3a RIGHT FEMUR, SUPERIOR VIEW B-30
FIGURE 9.3b RIGHT FEMUR, INFERIOR VIEW B-30
FIGURE 9.4a RIGHT TIBIA AND FIBULA, ANTERIOR VIEWS B-31
FIGURE 9.4b RIGHT TIBIA, SUPERIOR VIEW B-31
FIGURE 9.4c RIGHT TIBIA AND FIBULA, DISTAL, INFERIOR VIEW B-31
FIGURE 9.4d THE TIBIA AND FIBULA, POSTERIOR VIEWS B-31
FIGURE 9.5a RIGHT FOOT, SUPERIOR (DORSAL) VIEW B-32
FIGURE 9.5b RIGHT FOOT, INFERIOR (PLANTAR) VIEW B-32
FIGURE 9.5c RIGHT FOOT, LATERAL VIEW B-33

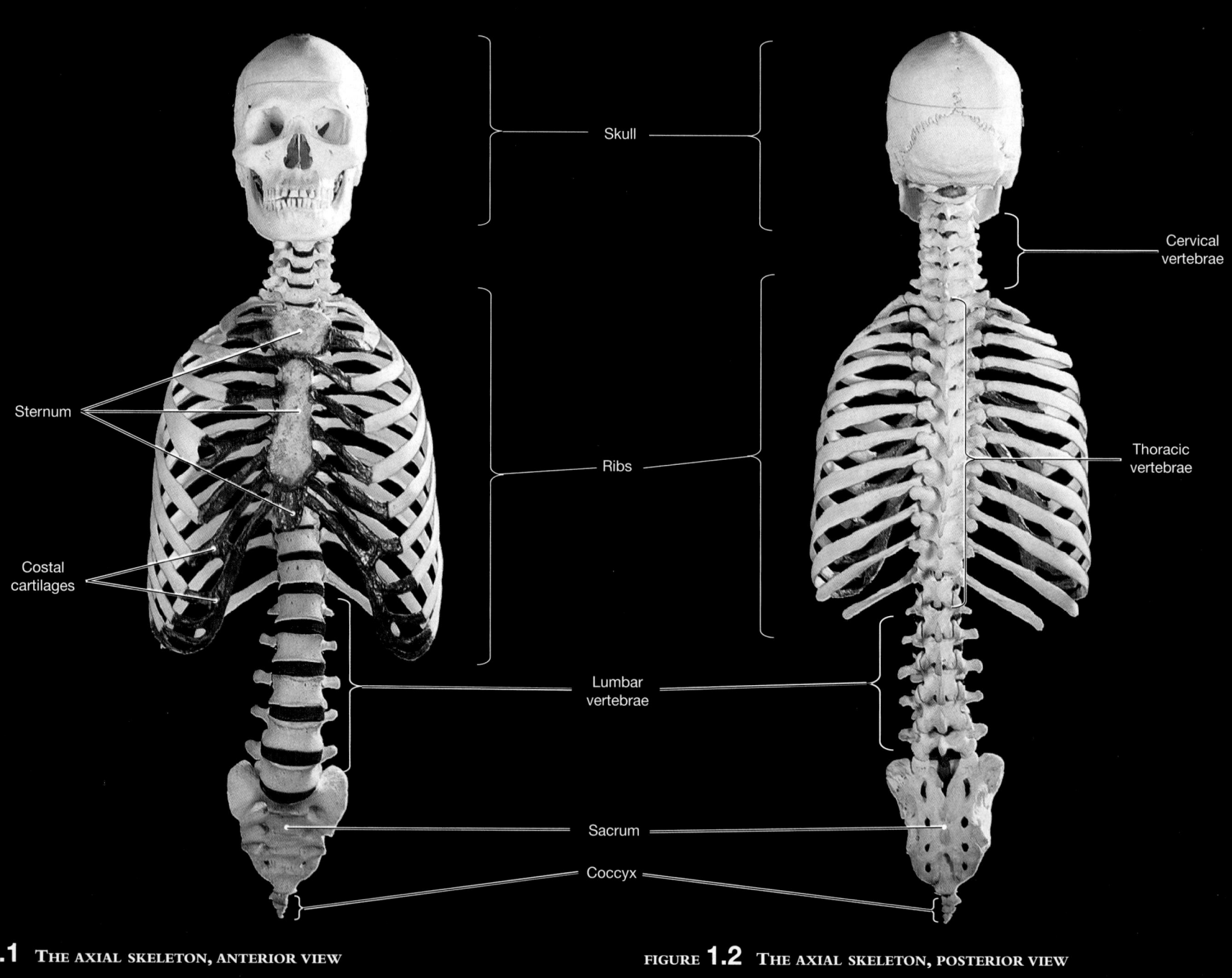

Skull

Cervical
vertebrae

Sternum

Ribs

Thoracic
vertebrae

Costal
cartilages

Lumbar
vertebrae

Sacrum

Coccyx

FIGURE **1.1** THE AXIAL SKELETON, ANTERIOR VIEW

FIGURE **1.2** THE AXIAL SKELETON, POSTERIOR VIEW

FIGURE **2.1** THE
SKELETON, ANTERIOR
VIEW

FIGURE **2.2** THE
SKELETON,
POSTERIOR VIEW

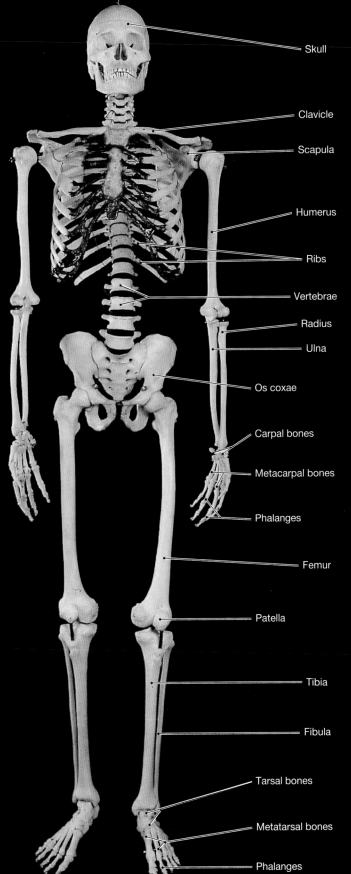

Skull

Clavicle

Scapula

Humerus

Ribs

Vertebrae

Radius

Ulna

Os coxae

Carpal bones

Metacarpal bones

Phalanges

Femur

Patella

Tibia

Fibula

Tarsal bones

Metatarsal bones

Phalanges

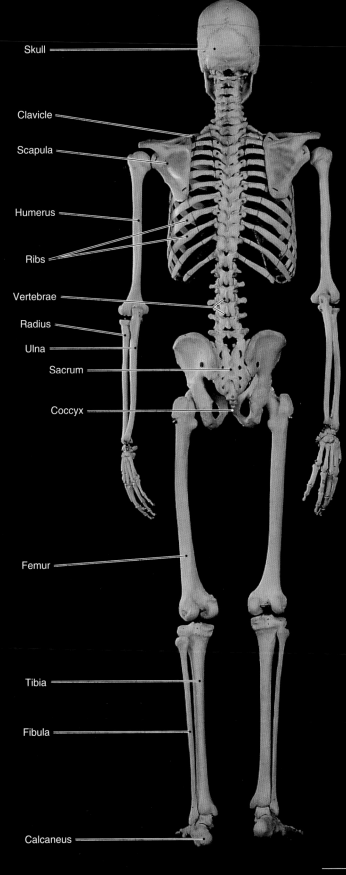

Skull

Clavicle

Scapula

Humerus

Ribs

Vertebrae

Radius

Ulna

Sacrum

Coccyx

Femur

Tibia

Fibula

Calcaneus

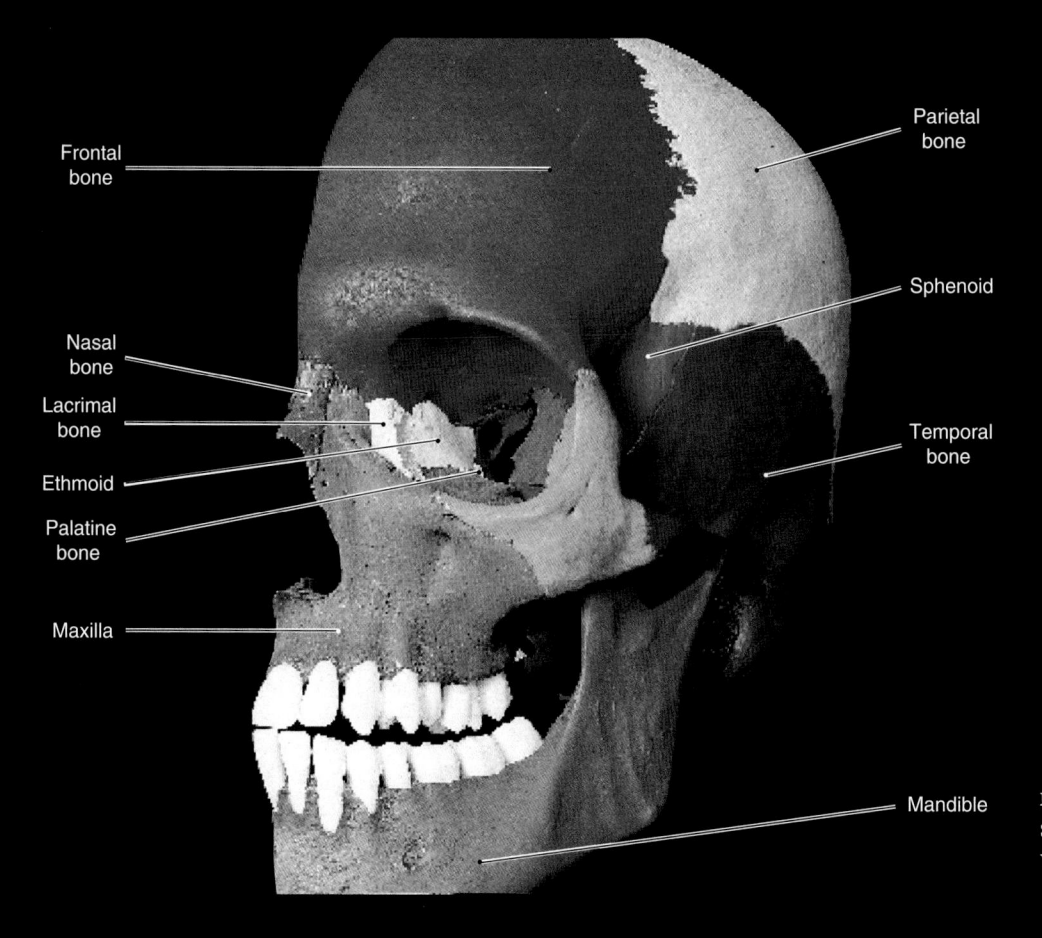

Frontal
bone

Parietal
bone

Sphenoid

Nasal
bone

Lacrimal
bone

Temporal
bone

Ethmoid

Palatine
bone

Maxilla

Mandible

FIGURE **3.1** PAINTED
SKULL, ANTEROLATERAL
VIEW

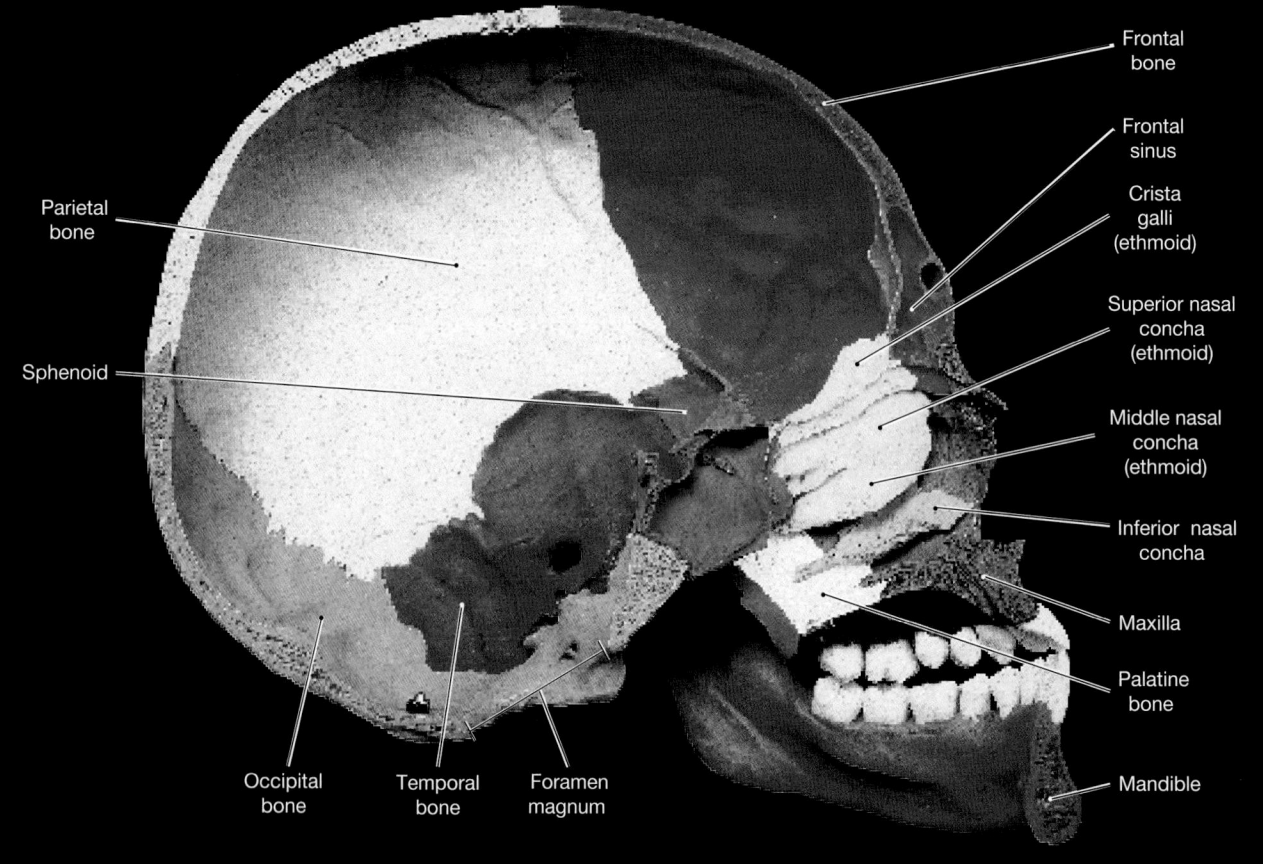

Parietal
bone

Frontal
bone

Frontal
sinus

Crista
galli
(ethmoid)

Superior nasal
concha
(ethmoid)

Sphenoid

Middle nasal
concha
(ethmoid)

Inferior nasal
concha

Maxilla

Palatine
bone

Occipital
bone

Temporal
bone

Foramen
magnum

Mandible

FIGURE **3.2** PAINTED
SKULL, MEDIAL VIEW

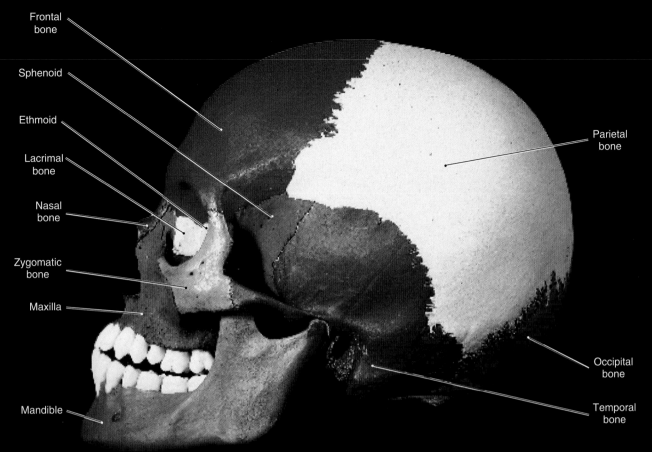

Frontal
bone

Sphenoid

Ethmoid

Lacrimal
bone

Nasal
bone

Zygomatic
bone

Maxilla

Mandible

Parietal
bone

Occipital
bone

Temporal
bone

FIGURE **3.3** PAINTED
SKULL, LATERAL VIEW

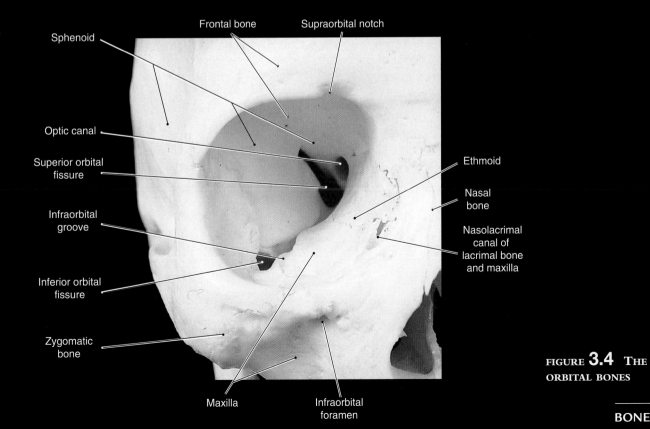

Sphenoid

Optic canal

Superior orbital
fissure

Infraorbital
groove

Inferior orbital
fissure

Zygomatic
bone

Frontal bone   Supraorbital notch

Ethmoid

Nasal
bone

Nasolacrimal
canal of
lacrimal bone
and maxilla

Maxilla

Infraorbital
foramen

FIGURE **3.4** THE
ORBITAL BONES

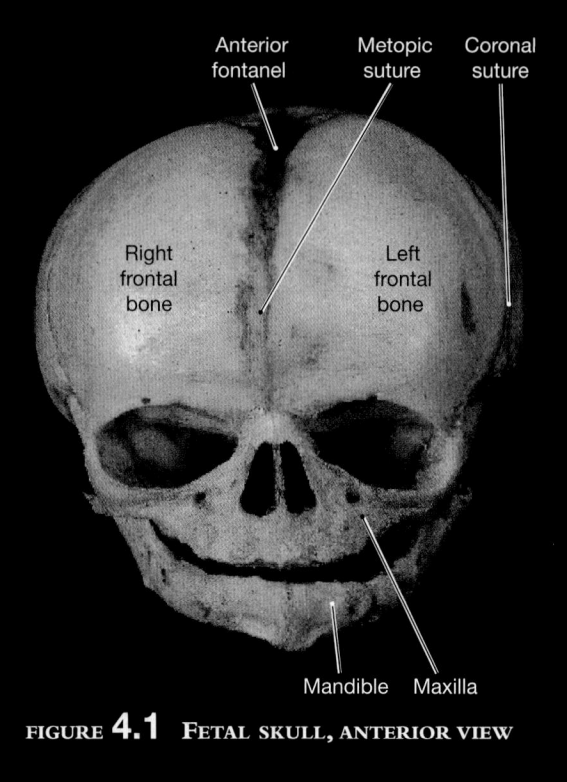

Anterior fontanel   Metopic suture   Coronal suture

Right frontal bone   Left frontal bone

Mandible   Maxilla

FIGURE **4.1** FETAL SKULL, ANTERIOR VIEW

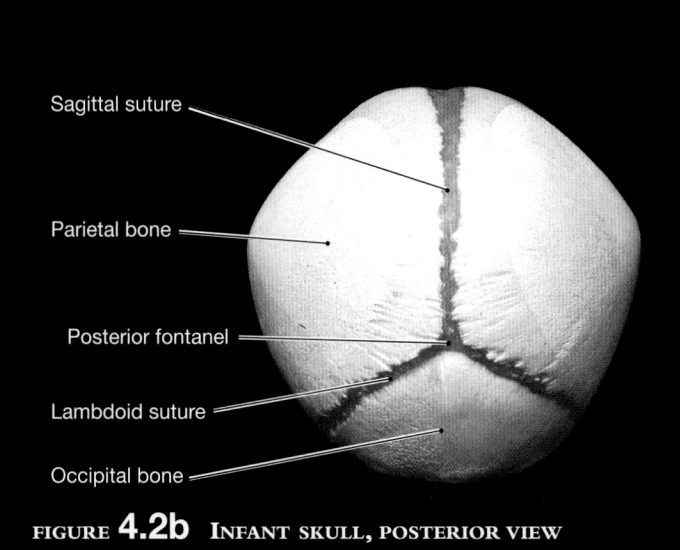

Sagittal suture

Parietal bone

Anterior fontanel

Coronal suture

Frontal bone

Metopic suture

FIGURE **4.2a** INFANT SKULL, ANTEROSUPERIOR VIEW

Sagittal suture

Parietal bone

Posterior fontanel

Lambdoid suture

Occipital bone

FIGURE **4.2b** INFANT SKULL, POSTERIOR VIEW

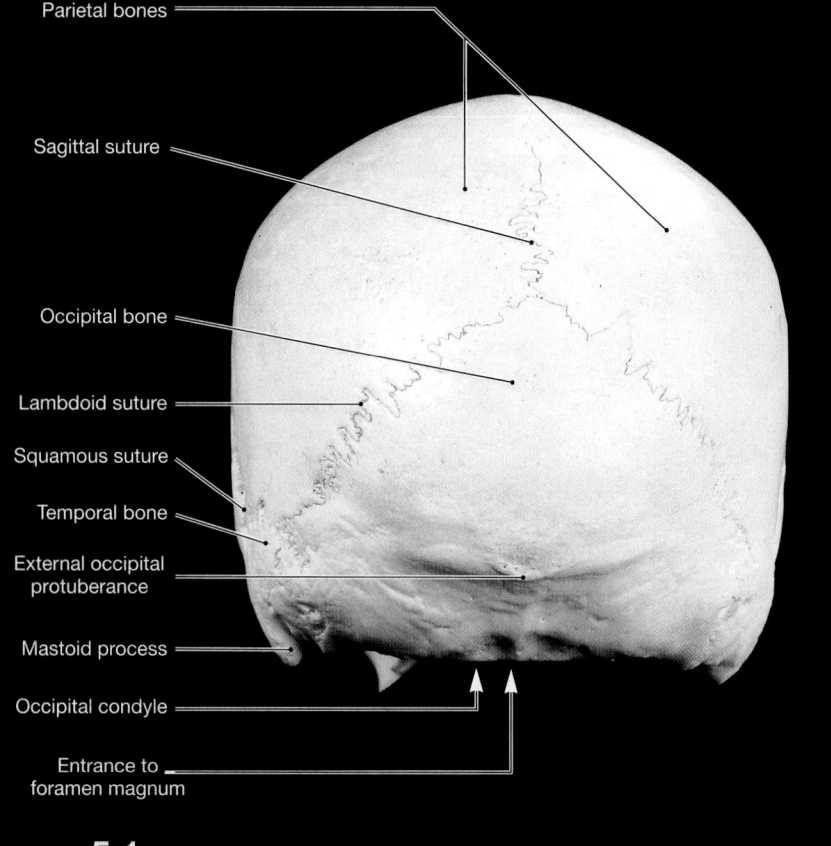

Parietal bones

Sagittal suture

Occipital bone

Lambdoid suture

Squamous suture

Temporal bone

External occipital protuberance

Mastoid process

Occipital condyle

Entrance to foramen magnum

FIGURE **5.1a** ADULT SKULL, POSTERIOR VIEW

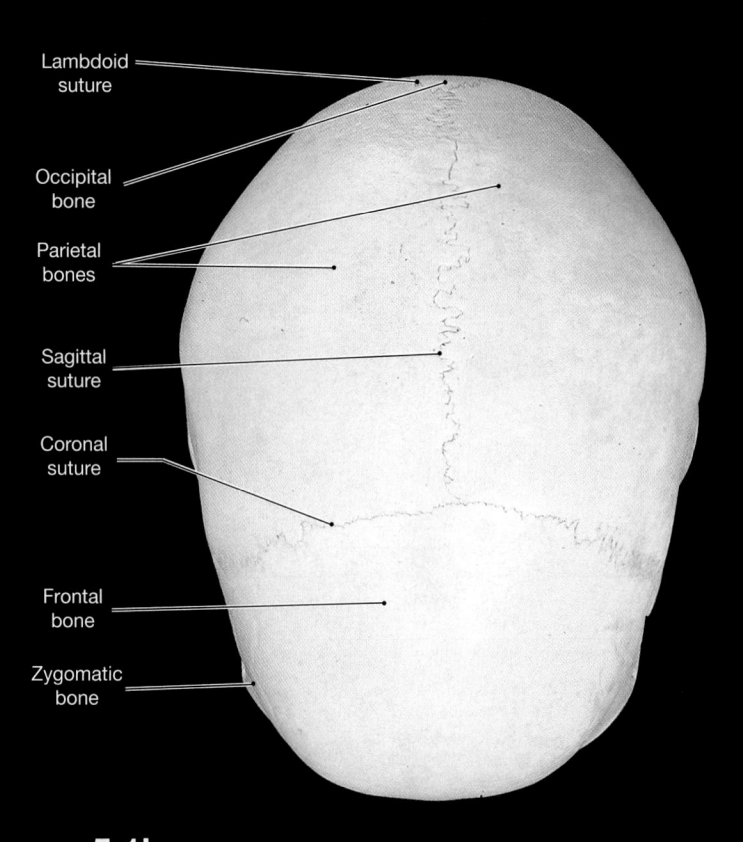

Lambdoid suture

Occipital bone

Parietal bones

Sagittal suture

Coronal suture

Frontal bone

Zygomatic bone

FIGURE **5.1b** ADULT SKULL, SUPERIOR VIEW

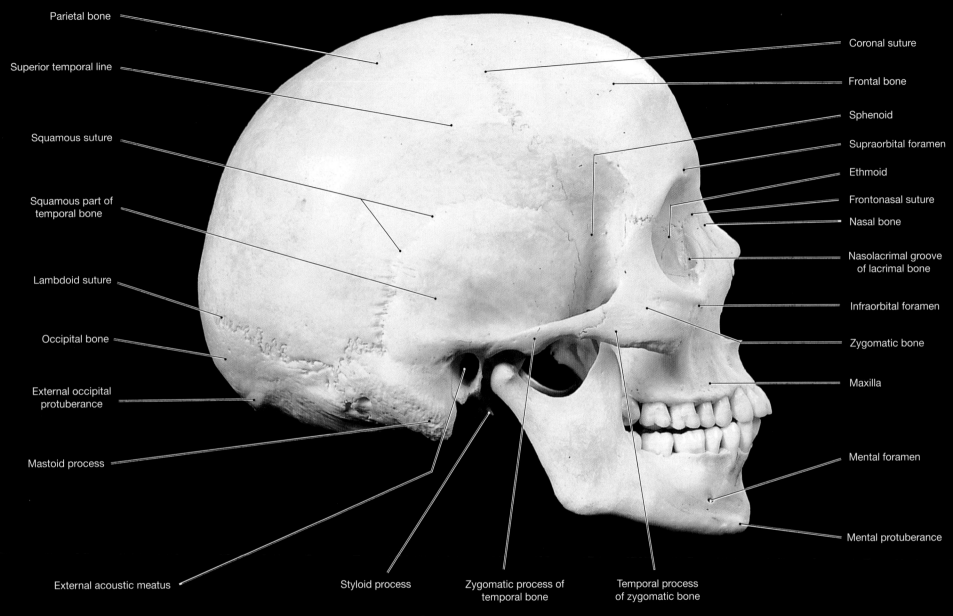

Parietal bone

Superior temporal line

Squamous suture

Squamous part of
temporal bone

Lambdoid suture

Occipital bone

External occipital
protuberance

Mastoid process

External acoustic meatus

Styloid process

Zygomatic process of
temporal bone

Temporal process
of zygomatic bone

Coronal suture

Frontal bone

Sphenoid

Supraorbital foramen

Ethmoid

Frontonasal suture

Nasal bone

Nasolacrimal groove
of lacrimal bone

Infraorbital foramen

Zygomatic bone

Maxilla

Mental foramen

Mental protuberance

FIGURE **5.2** ADULT SKULL, LATERAL VIEW

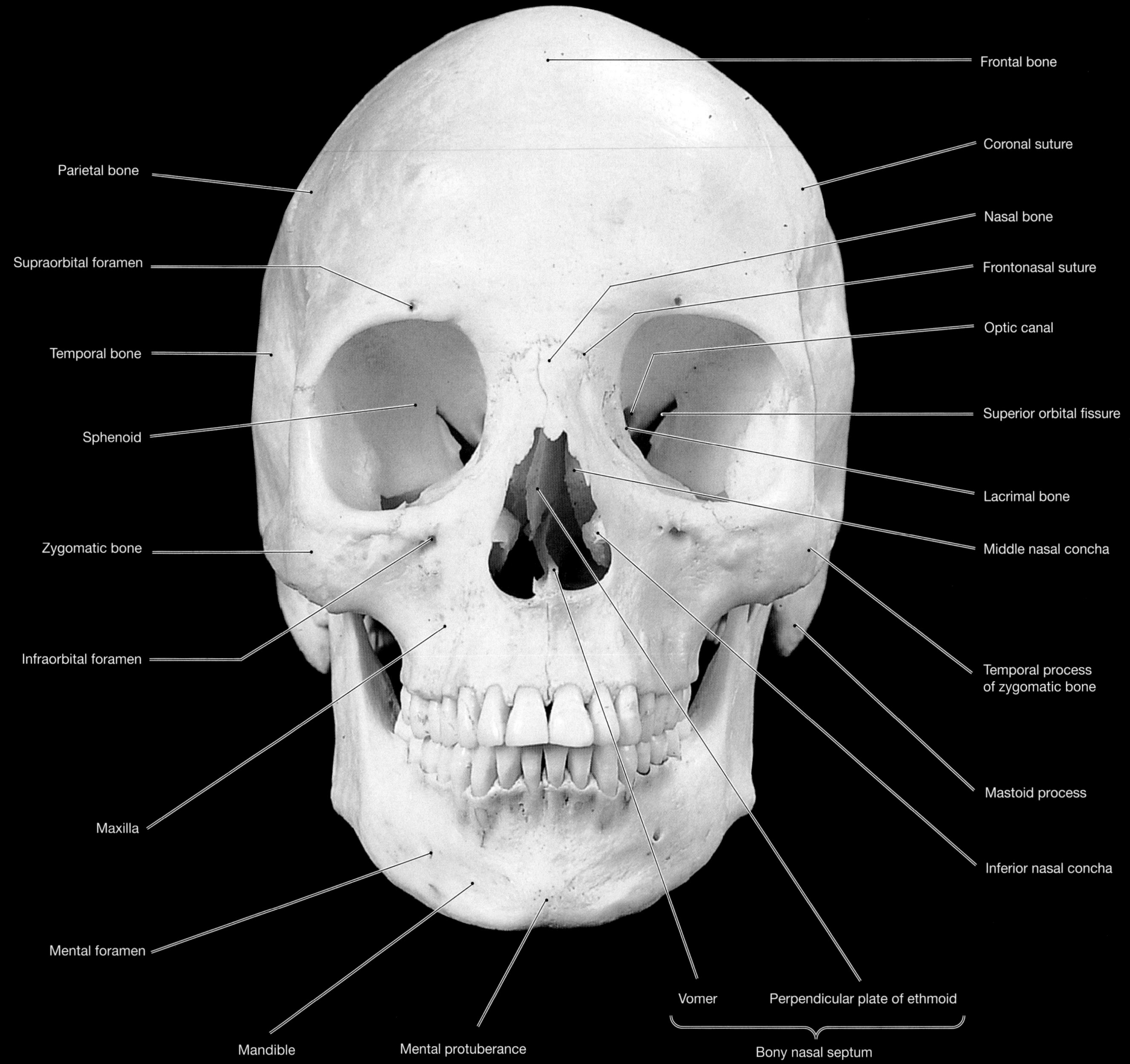

Frontal bone

Coronal suture

Parietal bone

Nasal bone

Supraorbital foramen

Frontonasal suture

Temporal bone

Optic canal

Sphenoid

Superior orbital fissure

Zygomatic bone

Lacrimal bone

Middle nasal concha

Infraorbital foramen

Temporal process
of zygomatic bone

Maxilla

Mastoid process

Inferior nasal concha

Mental foramen

Mandible

Mental protuberance

Vomer

Perpendicular plate of ethmoid

Bony nasal septum

FIGURE **5.3** ADULT SKULL, ANTERIOR VIEW

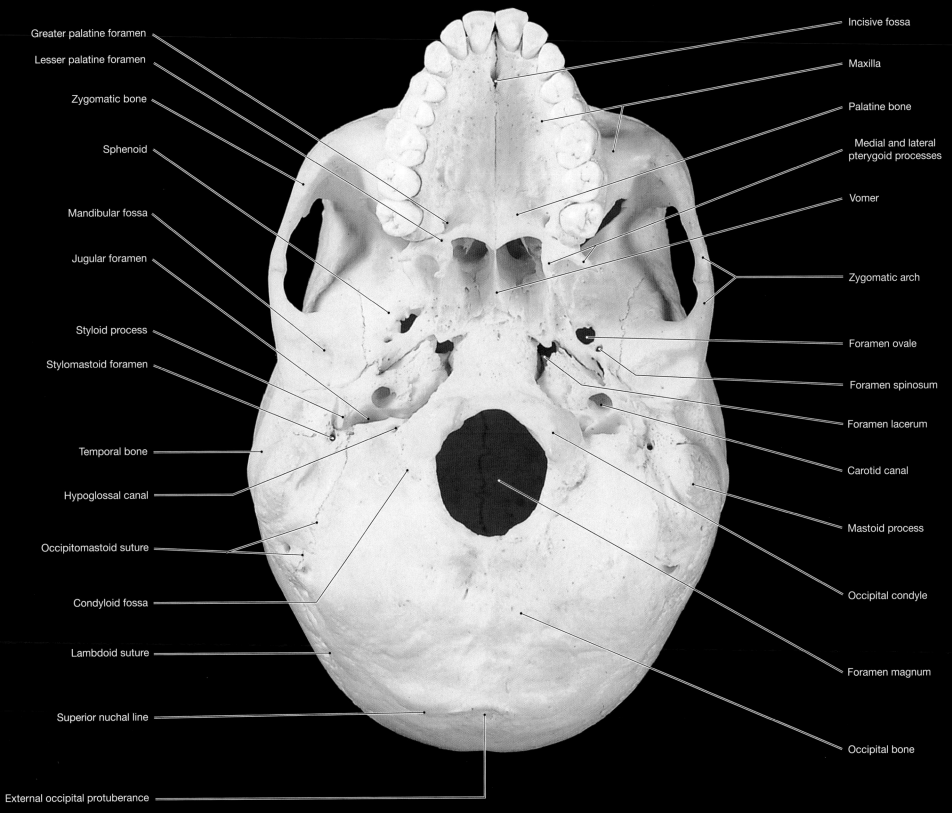

Greater palatine foramen
Lesser palatine foramen
Zygomatic bone
Sphenoid
Mandibular fossa
Jugular foramen
Styloid process
Stylomastoid foramen
Temporal bone
Hypoglossal canal
Occipitomastoid suture
Condyloid fossa
Lambdoid suture
Superior nuchal line
External occipital protuberance

Incisive fossa
Maxilla
Palatine bone
Medial and lateral pterygoid processes
Vomer
Zygomatic arch
Foramen ovale
Foramen spinosum
Foramen lacerum
Carotid canal
Mastoid process
Occipital condyle
Foramen magnum
Occipital bone

FIGURE **5.4** ADULT SKULL, INFERIOR VIEW, MANDIBLE REMOVED

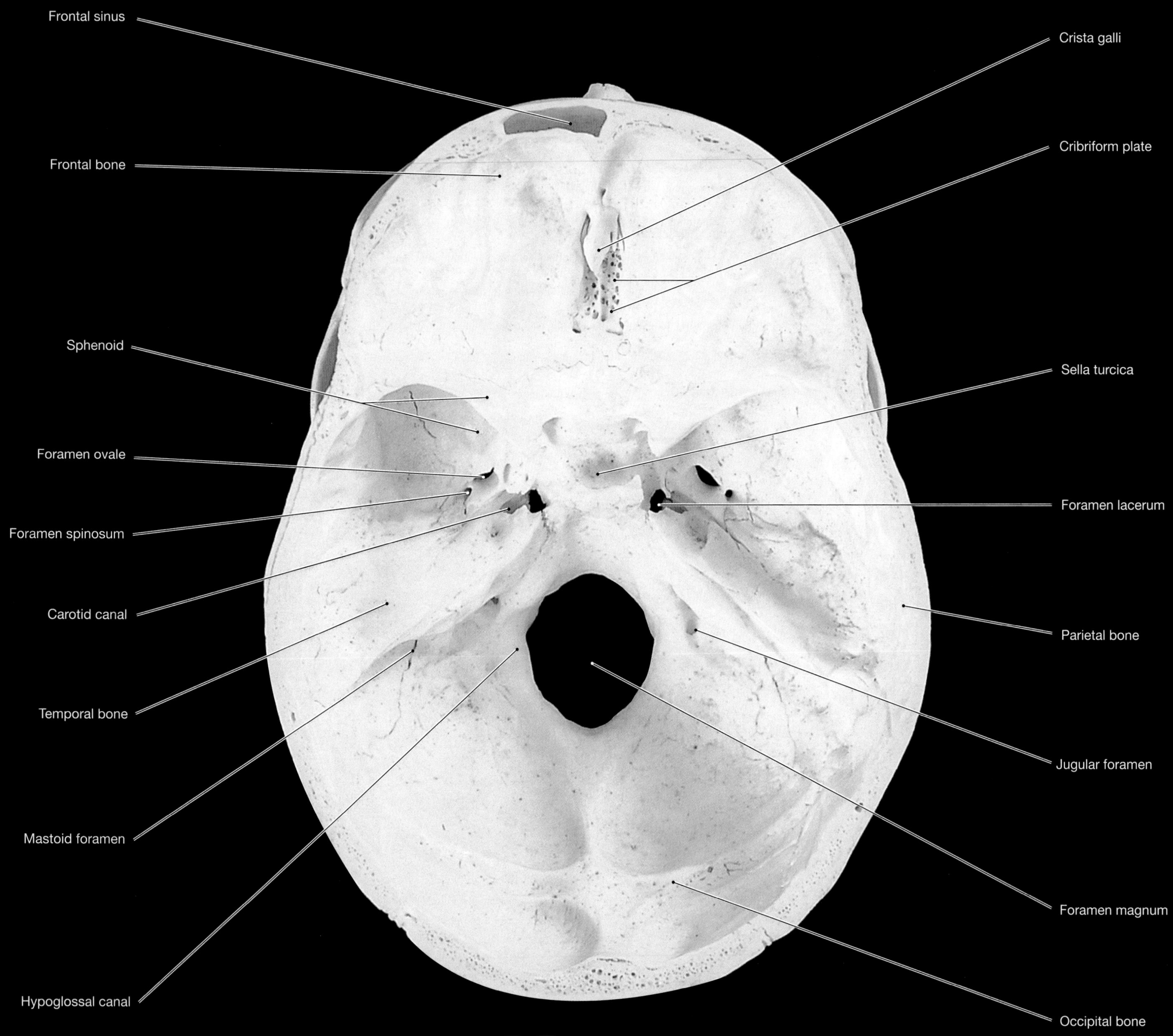

FIGURE 5.5 ADULT SKULL: HORIZONTAL SECTION

Occipital bone

Foramen magnum

Jugular foramen

Parietal bone

Foramen lacerum

Sella turcica

Cribriform plate

Crista galli

Hypoglossal canal

Mastoid foramen

Temporal bone

Carotid canal

Foramen spinosum

Foramen ovale

Sphenoid

Frontal bone

Frontal sinus

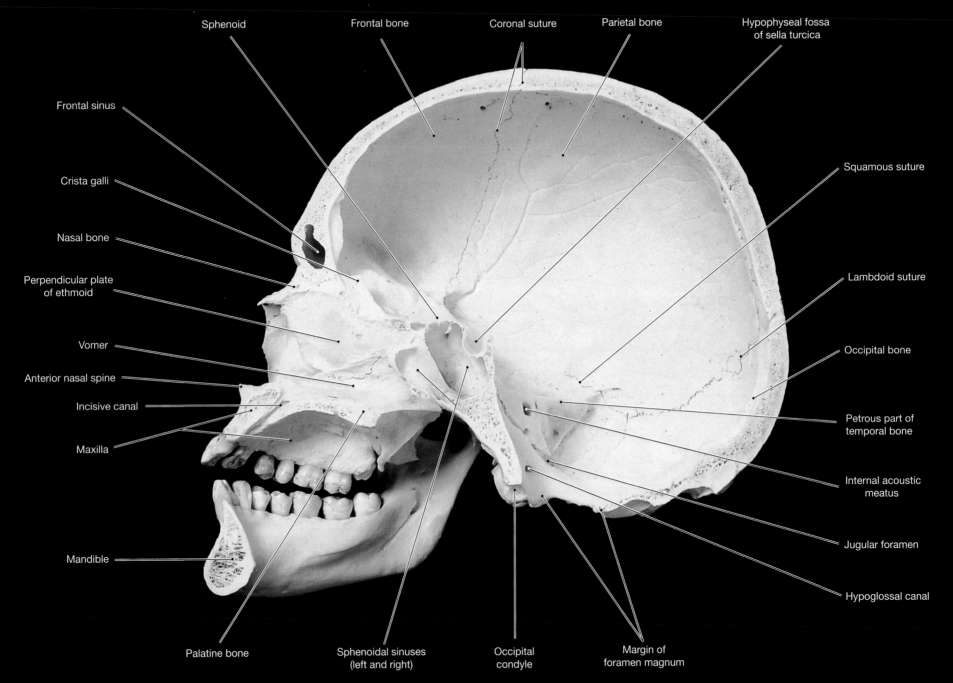

Sphenoid

Frontal bone

Coronal suture

Parietal bone

Hypophyseal fossa
of sella turcica

Frontal sinus

Squamous suture

Crista galli

Nasal bone

Lambdoid suture

Perpendicular plate
of ethmoid

Vomer

Occipital bone

Anterior nasal spine

Incisive canal

Petrous part of
temporal bone

Maxilla

Internal acoustic
meatus

Mandible

Jugular foramen

Hypoglossal canal

Palatine bone

Sphenoidal sinuses
(left and right)

Occipital
condyle

Margin of
foramen magnum

FIGURE **5.6** ADULT SKULL, SAGITTAL SECTION

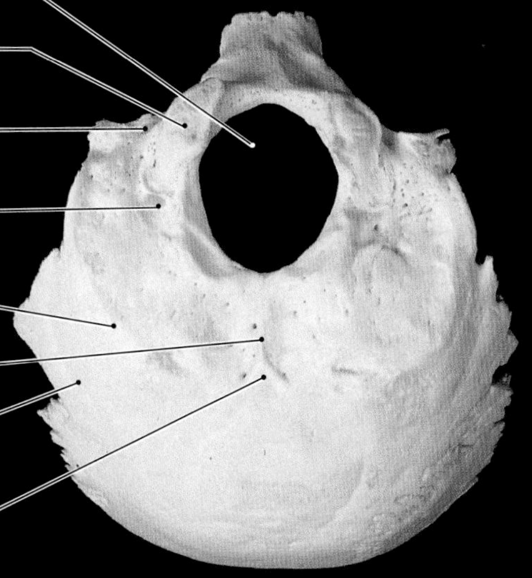

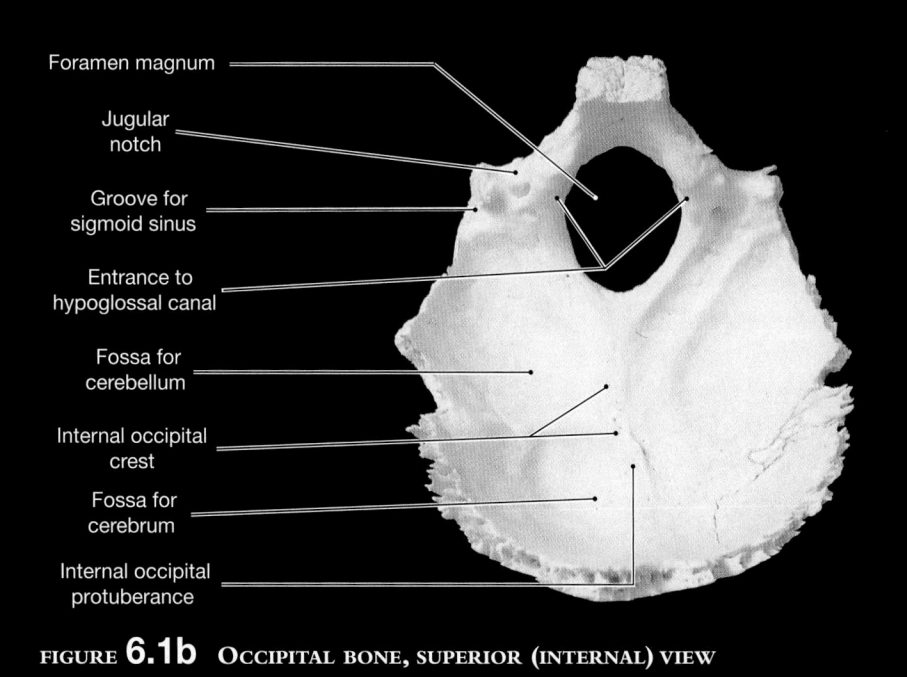

Foramen magnum

Occipital
condyle

Hypoglossal
canal

Condyloid
fossa

Inferior nuchal
line

External
occipital
crest

Superior
nuchal
line

External occipital
protuberance

FIGURE **6.1a** OCCIPITAL BONE, INFERIOR (EXTERNAL) VIEW

Foramen magnum

Jugular
notch

Groove for
sigmoid sinus

Entrance to
hypoglossal canal

Fossa for
cerebellum

Internal occipital
crest

Fossa for
cerebrum

Internal occipital
protuberance

FIGURE **6.1b** OCCIPITAL BONE, SUPERIOR (INTERNAL) VIEW

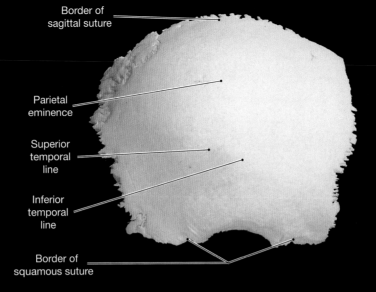

Border of
sagittal suture

Parietal
eminence

Superior
temporal
line

Inferior
temporal
line

Border of
squamous suture

FIGURE **6.2** PARIETAL BONE, LATERAL VIEW

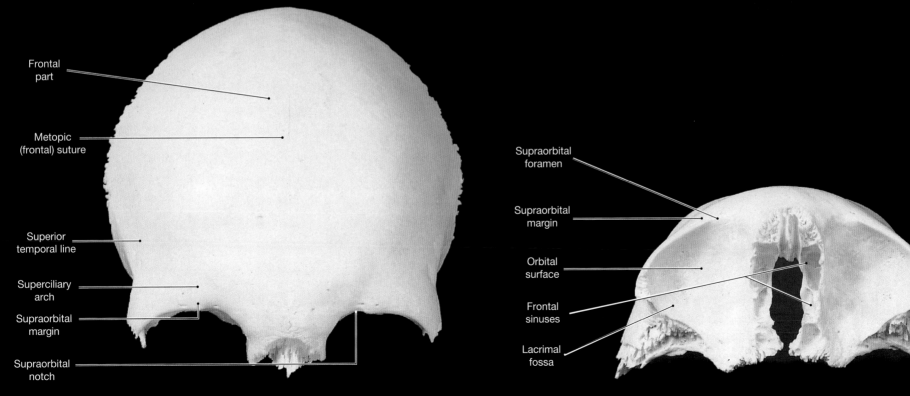

Frontal
part

Metopic
(frontal) suture

Superior
temporal line

Superciliary
arch

Supraorbital
margin

Supraorbital
notch

FIGURE **6.3a** FRONTAL BONE, ANTERIOR VIEW

Supraorbital
foramen

Supraorbital
margin

Orbital
surface

Frontal
sinuses

Lacrimal
fossa

FIGURE **6.3b** FRONTAL BONE, INFERIOR VIEW

FIGURE 6.4b TEMPORAL BONE RIGHT TEMPORAL BONE MEDIAL VIEW

FIGURE 6.4a TEMPORAL BONE RIGHT TEMPORAL BONE LATERAL VIEW

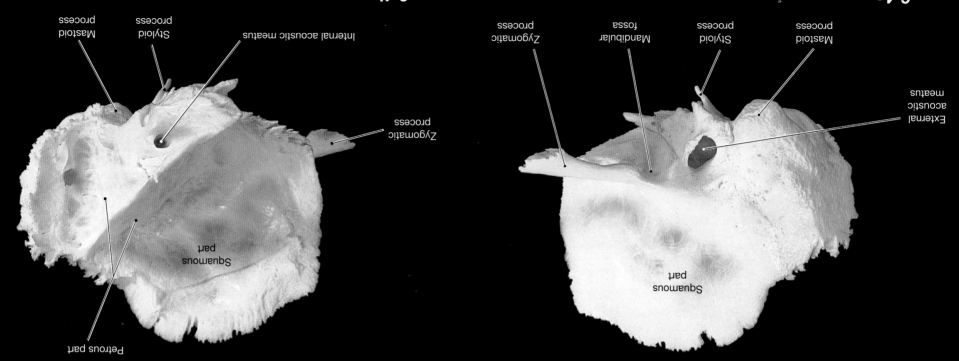

Mastoid process — Styloid process — Internal acoustic meatus — Zygomatic process — Squamous part — Petrous part

Zygomatic process — Mandibular fossa — Styloid process — Mastoid process — External acoustic meatus — Squamous part

FIGURE 6.3C FRONTAL BONE, POSTERIOR (INTERNAL) VIEW

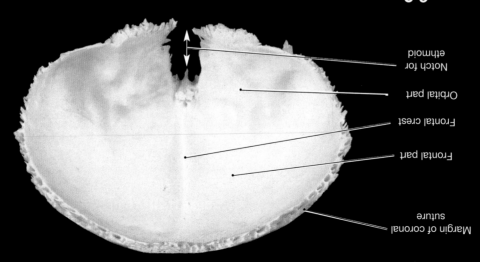

Notch for ethmoid — Orbital part — Frontal crest — Frontal part — Margin of coronal suture

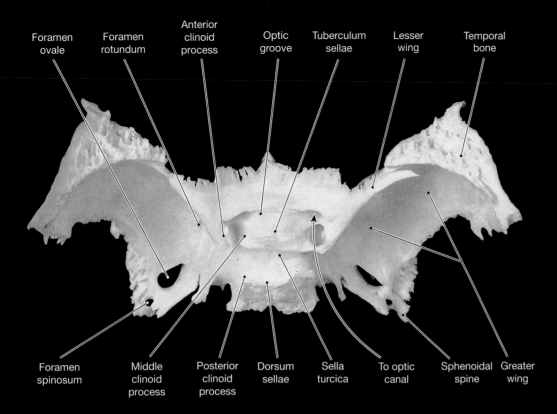

Foramen ovale
Foramen rotundum
Anterior clinoid process
Optic groove
Tuberculum sellae
Lesser wing
Temporal bone

Foramen spinosum
Middle clinoid process
Posterior clinoid process
Dorsum sellae
Sella turcica
To optic canal
Sphenoidal spine
Greater wing

FIGURE 6.5a SPHENOID, SUPERIOR SURFACE

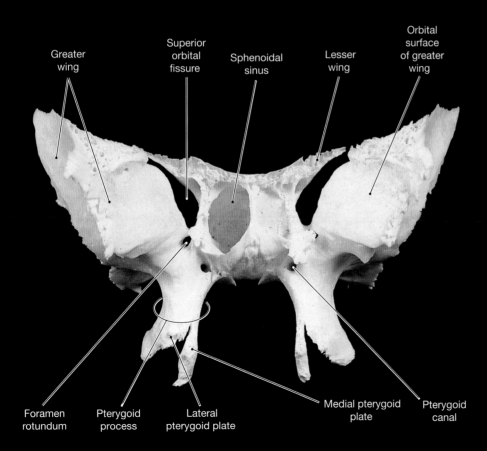

Greater wing
Superior orbital fissure
Sphenoidal sinus
Lesser wing
Orbital surface of greater wing

Foramen rotundum
Pterygoid process
Lateral pterygoid plate
Medial pterygoid plate
Pterygoid canal

FIGURE 6.5b SPHENOID, ANTERIOR SURFACE

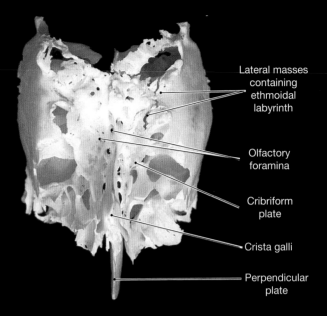

Lateral masses containing ethmoidal labyrinth
Olfactory foramina
Cribriform plate
Crista galli
Perpendicular plate

FIGURE 6.6a ETHMOID, SUPERIOR VIEW

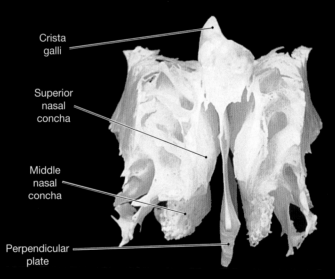

Crista galli
Superior nasal concha
Middle nasal concha
Perpendicular plate

FIGURE 6.6b ETHMOID, POSTERIOR VIEW

BONE IMAGES **B-15**

FIGURE 6.8b RIGHT MAXILLA, MEDIAL VIEW

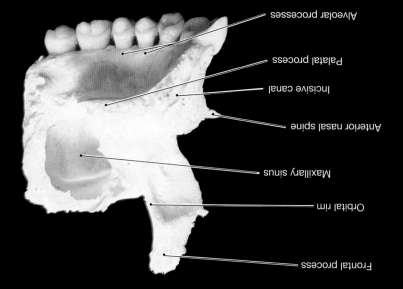

Alveolar processes

Palatal process

Incisive canal

Anterior nasal spine

Maxillary sinus

Orbital rim

Frontal process

FIGURE 6.7 CRANIAL FOSSAE, SUPERIOR VIEW

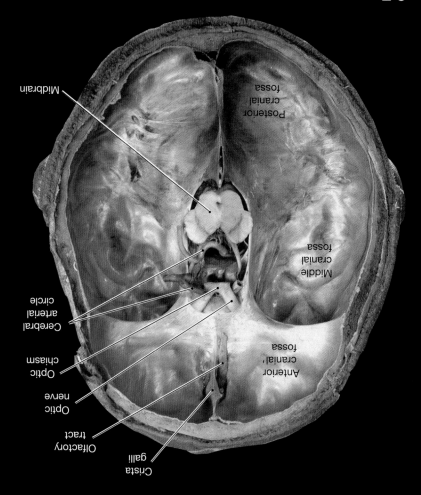

Midbrain

Posterior cranial fossa

Middle cranial fossa

Cerebral arterial circle

Optic chiasm

Anterior cranial fossa

Optic nerve

Olfactory tract

Crista galli

FIGURE 6.8a RIGHT MAXILLA, LATERAL VIEW

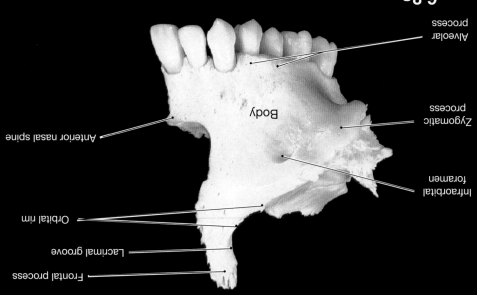
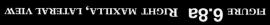

Alveolar process

Body

Zygomatic process

Anterior nasal spine

Infraorbital foramen

Orbital rim

Lacrimal groove

Frontal process

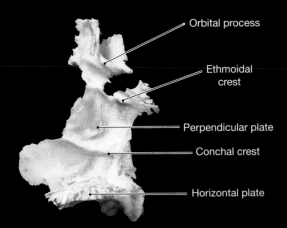

Orbital process

Ethmoidal crest

Perpendicular plate

Conchal crest

Horizontal plate

FIGURE **6.9a** RIGHT PALATINE BONE, MEDIAL VIEW

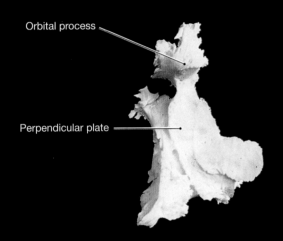

Orbital process

Perpendicular plate

FIGURE **6.9b** RIGHT PALATINE BONE, LATERAL VIEW

FIGURE **6.10a**
MANDIBLE, LATERAL VIEW

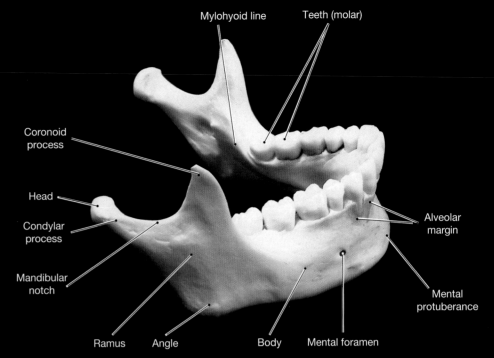

Mylohyoid line

Teeth (molar)

Coronoid process

Head

Condylar process

Mandibular notch

Alveolar margin

Mental protuberance

Ramus   Angle   Body   Mental foramen

FIGURE **6.10b**
MANDIBLE, MEDIAL VIEW

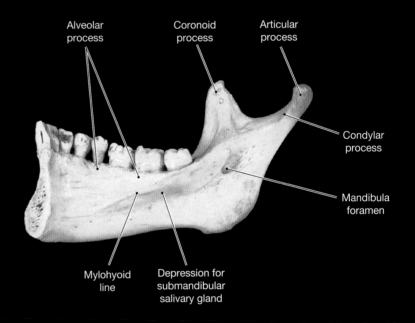

Alveolar process

Coronoid process

Articular process

Condylar process

Mandibula foramen

Mylohyoid line

Depression for submandibular salivary gland

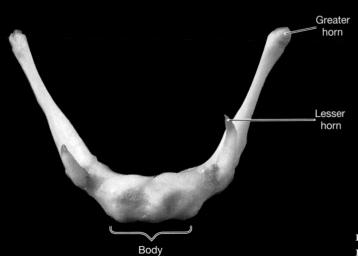

Greater horn

Lesser horn

Body

FIGURE **6.11** HYOID BONE, ANTERIOR VIEW

FIGURE 7.1 Vertebral column, lateral view

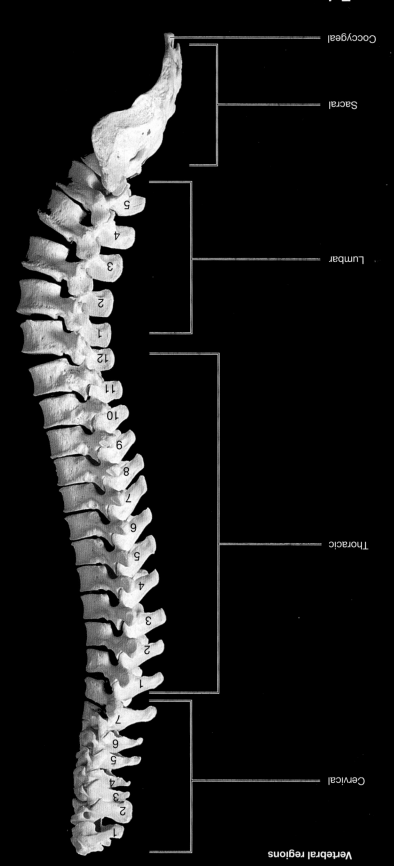

Coccygeal

Sacral

Lumbar

Thoracic

Cervical

Vertebral regions

FIGURE 7.2b Thoracic vertebrae, lateral view

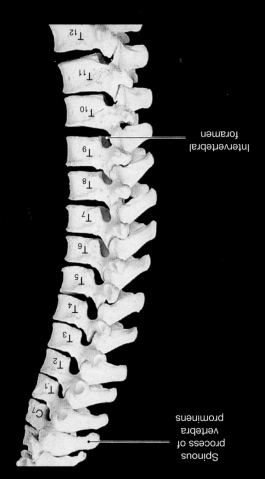

Intervertebral foramen

Spinous process of vertebra prominens

FIGURE 7.2a Cervical vertebrae, lateral view

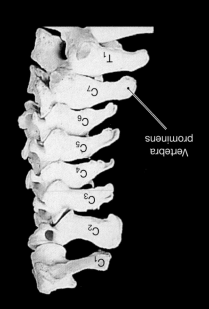

Vertebra prominens

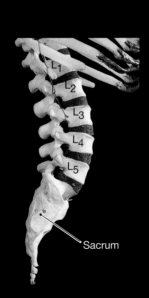

L-1
L-2
L-3
L-4
L-5

Sacrum

FIGURE **7.2c** LUMBAR VERTEBRAE, LATERAL VIEW

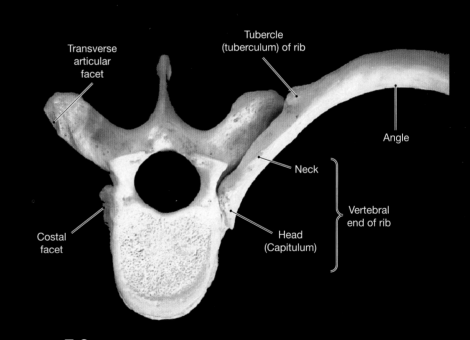

Transverse
articular
facet

Tubercle
(tuberculum) of rib

Angle

Neck

Vertebral
end of rib

Costal
facet

Head
(Capitulum)

FIGURE **7.3a** THORACIC VERTEBRA AND RIB, SUPERIOR VIEW

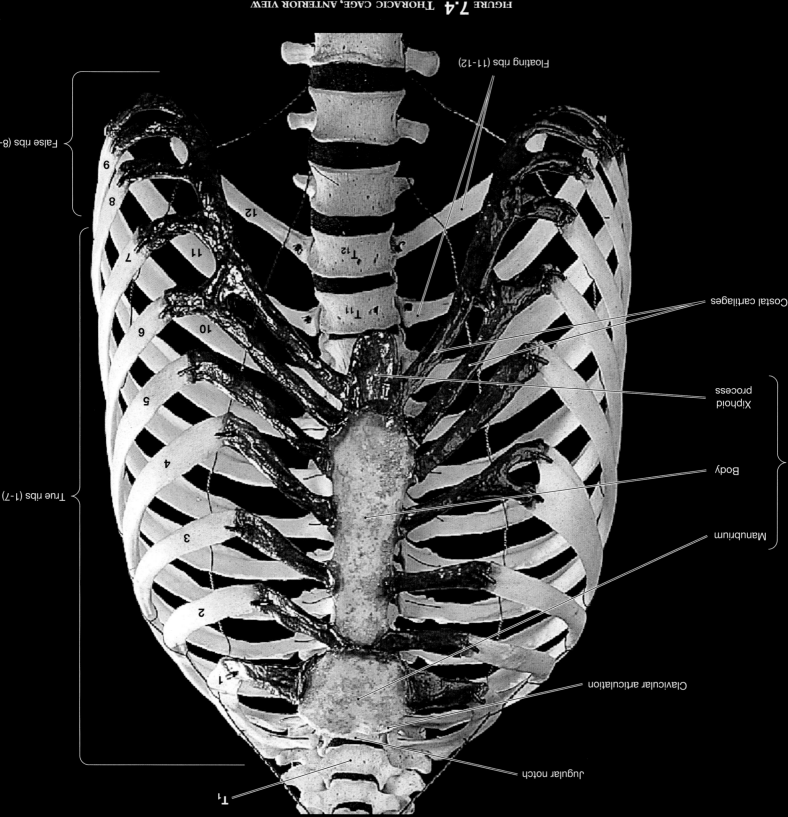

FIGURE 7.4 THORACIC CAGE, ANTERIOR VIEW

False ribs (8-

True ribs (1-7)

Floating ribs (11-12)

Costal cartilages

Xiphoid process

Body

Manubrium

Clavicular articulation

Jugular notch

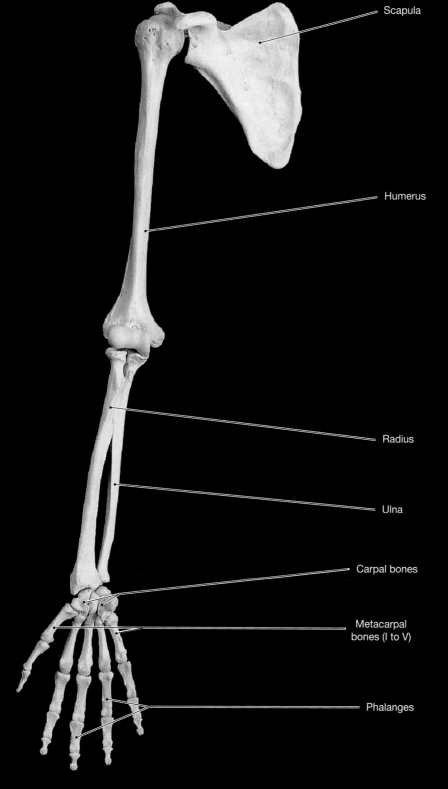

Scapula

Humerus

Radius

Ulna

Carpal bones

Metacarpal
bones (I to V)

Phalanges

FIGURE 8.1 PECTORAL GIRDLE AND RIGHT UPPER LIMB, ANTERIOR VIEW

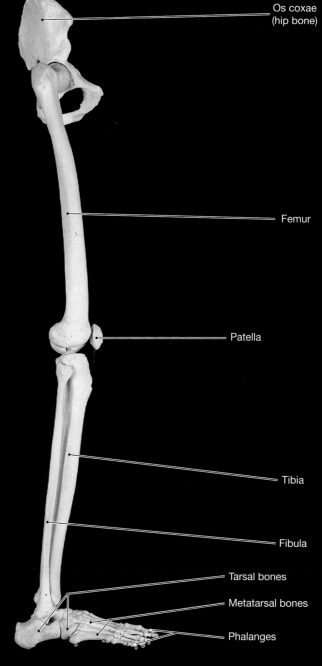

Os coxae
(hip bone)

Femur

Patella

Tibia

Fibula

Tarsal bones

Metatarsal bones

Phalanges

FIGURE 8.2 PELVIC GIRDLE AND RIGHT LOWER LIMB, LATERAL VIEW

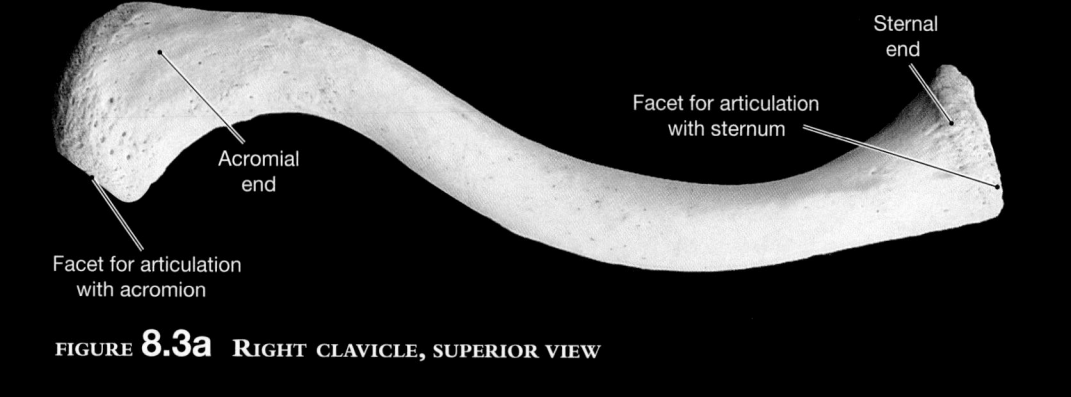

Sternal
end

Facet for articulation
with sternum

Acromial
end

Facet for articulation
with acromion

FIGURE **8.3a** RIGHT CLAVICLE, SUPERIOR VIEW

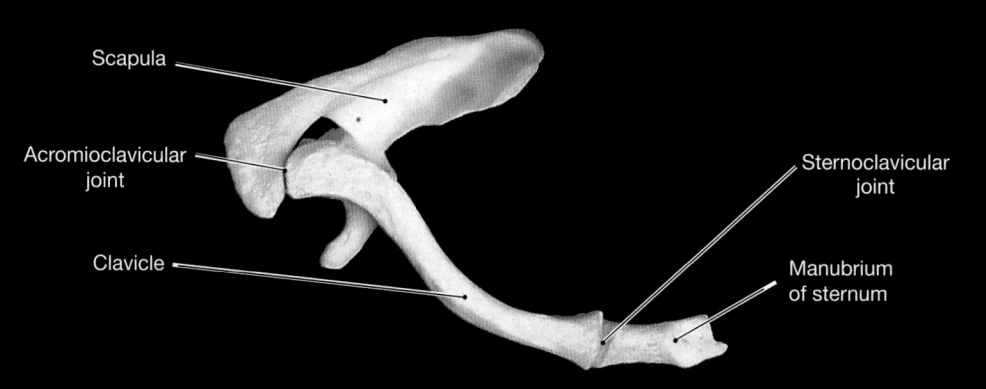

Scapula

Acromioclavicular
joint

Clavicle

Sternoclavicular
joint

Manubrium
of sternum

FIGURE **8.4** RIGHT PECTORAL GIRDLE, SUPERIOR VIEW

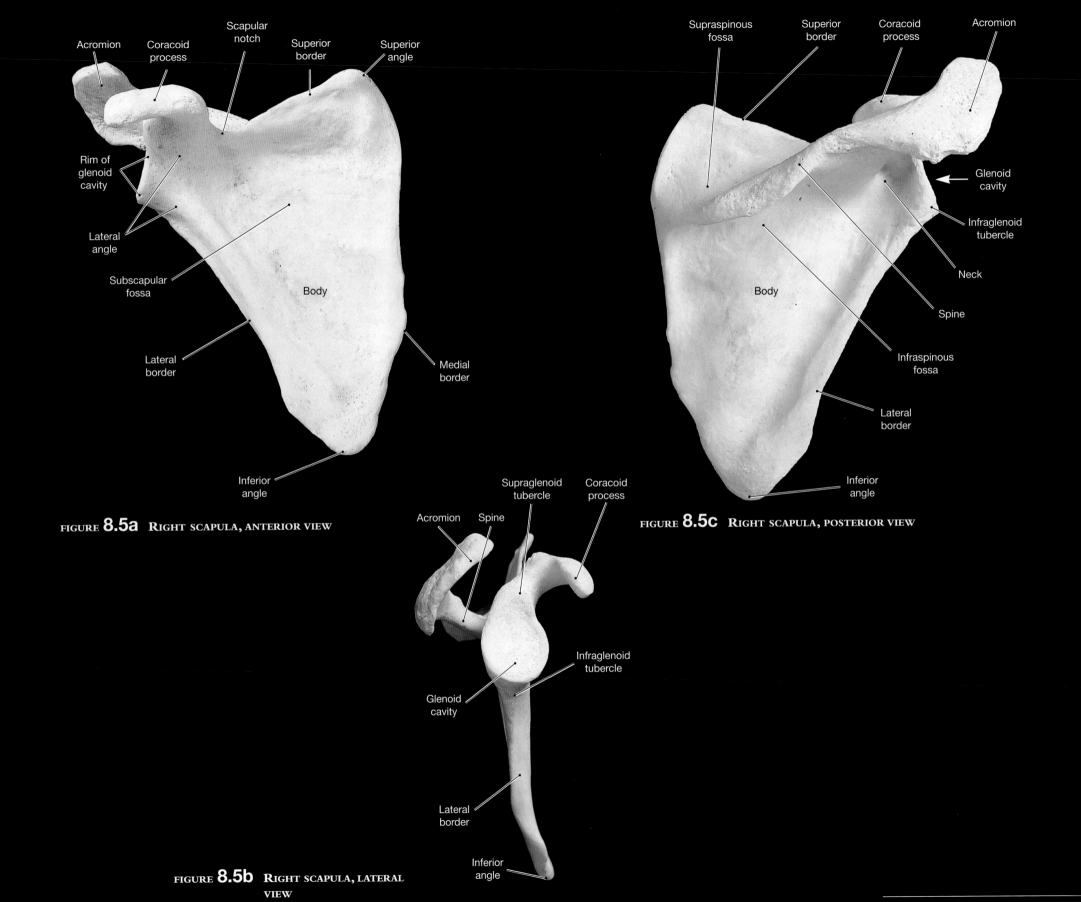

Acromion

Coracoid process

Scapular notch

Superior border

Superior angle

Rim of glenoid cavity

Lateral angle

Subscapular fossa

Body

Lateral border

Medial border

Inferior angle

FIGURE 8.5a RIGHT SCAPULA, ANTERIOR VIEW

Supraspinous fossa

Superior border

Coracoid process

Acromion

Glenoid cavity

Infraglenoid tubercle

Neck

Body

Spine

Infraspinous fossa

Lateral border

Inferior angle

FIGURE 8.5c RIGHT SCAPULA, POSTERIOR VIEW

Acromion

Spine

Supraglenoid tubercle

Coracoid process

Glenoid cavity

Infraglenoid tubercle

Lateral border

Inferior angle

FIGURE 8.5b RIGHT SCAPULA, LATERAL VIEW

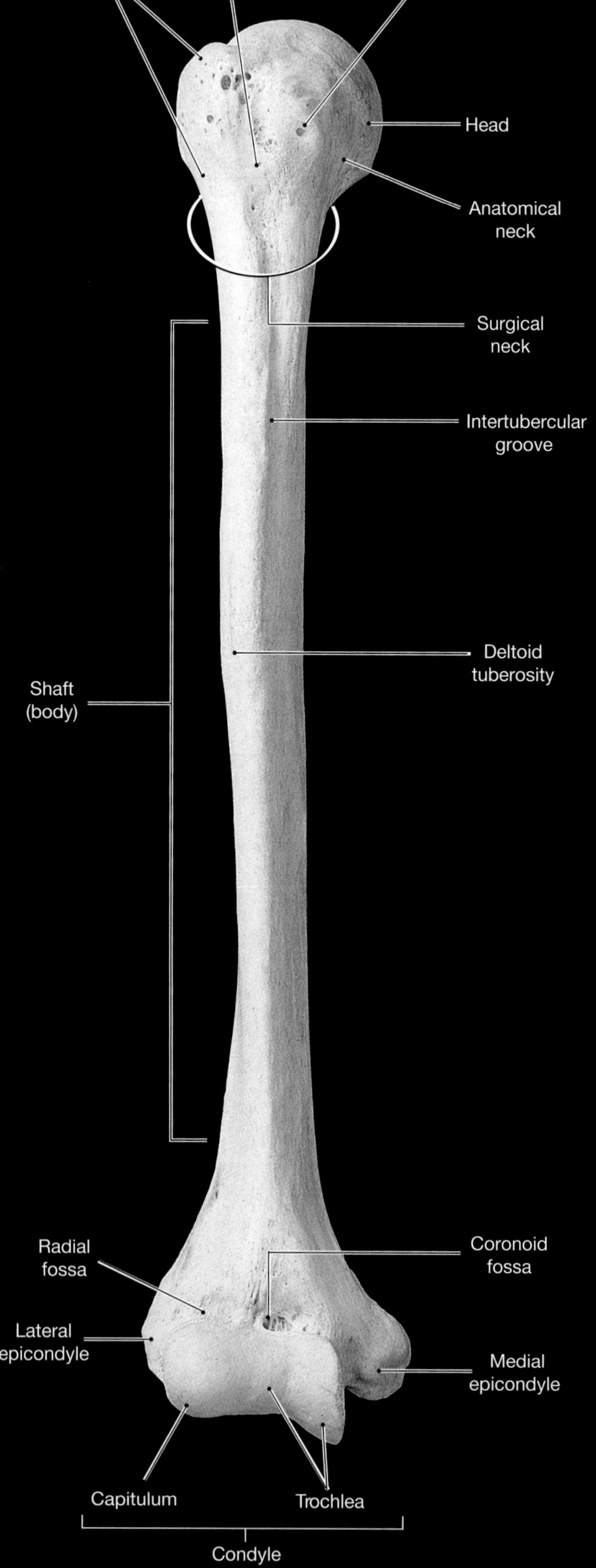

Head

Anatomical
neck

Surgical
neck

Intertubercular
groove

Shaft
(body)

Deltoid
tuberosity

Radial
fossa

Coronoid
fossa

Lateral
epicondyle

Medial
epicondyle

Capitulum

Trochlea

Condyle

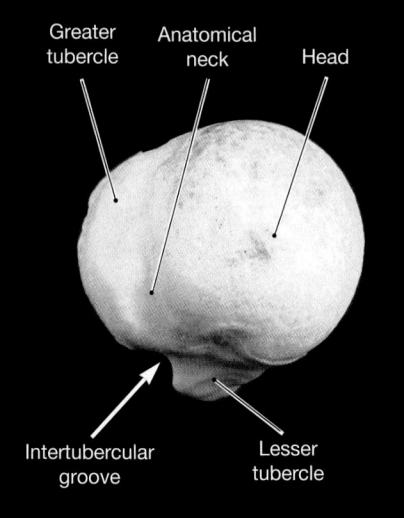

Greater
tubercle

Anatomical
neck

Head

Intertubercular
groove

Lesser
tubercle

FIGURE **8.6b** RIGHT HUMERUS, PROXIMAL, SUPERIOR VIEW

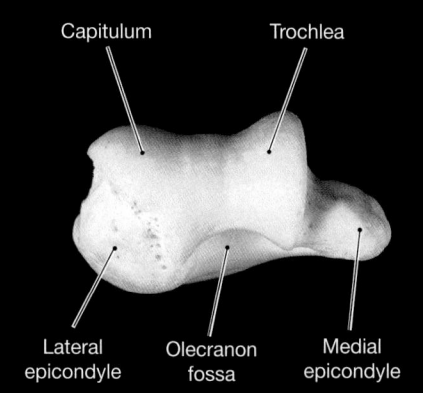

Capitulum

Trochlea

Lateral
epicondyle

Olecranon
fossa

Medial
epicondyle

FIGURE **8.6c** RIGHT HUMERUS, DISTAL, INFERIOR VIEW

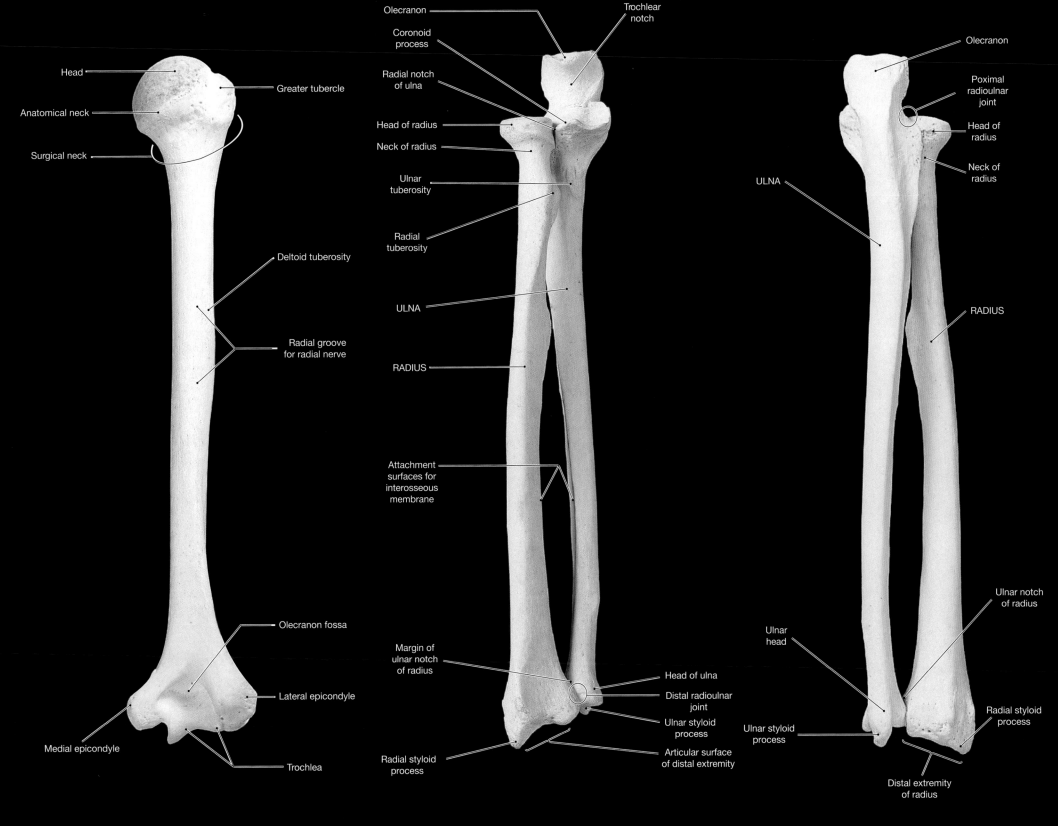

Head

Greater tubercle

Anatomical neck

Surgical neck

Deltoid tuberosity

Radial groove
for radial nerve

Olecranon fossa

Lateral epicondyle

Medial epicondyle

Trochlea

FIGURE 8.6d RIGHT HUMERUS, POSTERIOR VIEW

Olecranon

Coronoid
process

Trochlear
notch

Radial notch
of ulna

Head of radius

Neck of radius

Ulnar
tuberosity

Radial
tuberosity

ULNA

RADIUS

Attachment
surfaces for
interosseous
membrane

Margin of
ulnar notch
of radius

Head of ulna

Distal radioulnar
joint

Ulnar styloid
process

Articular surface
of distal extremity

Radial styloid
process

FIGURE 8.7a RIGHT RADIUS AND ULNA, ANTERIOR
VIEW

Olecranon

Poximal
radioulnar
joint

Head of
radius

Neck of
radius

ULNA

RADIUS

Ulnar notch
of radius

Ulnar
head

Radial styloid
process

Ulnar styloid
process

Distal extremity
of radius

FIGURE 8.7b RIGHT RADIUS AND ULNA,
POSTERIOR VIEW

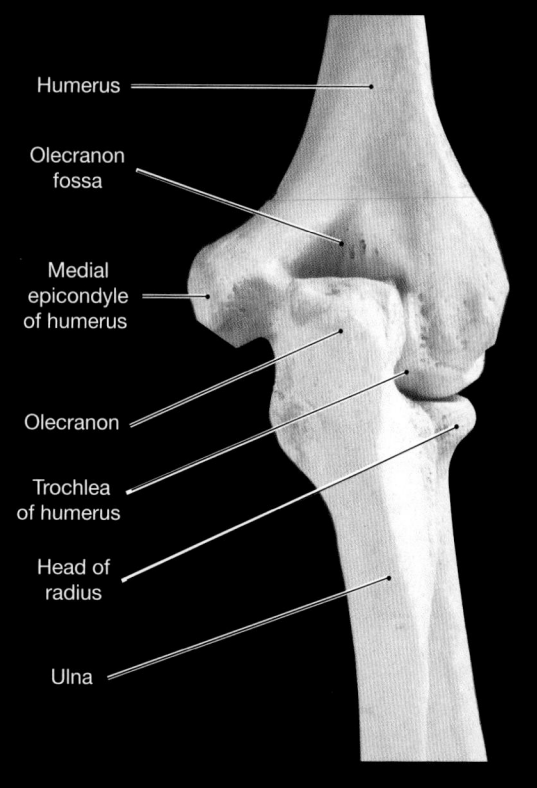

Humerus

Olecranon
fossa

Medial
epicondyle
of humerus

Olecranon

Trochlea
of humerus

Head of
radius

Ulna

FIGURE **8.8a** RIGHT ELBOW JOINT, POSTERIOR VIEW

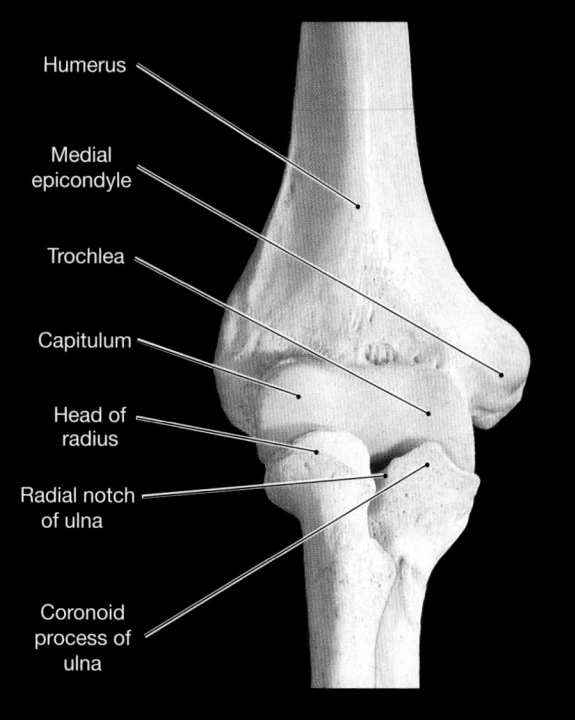

Humerus

Medial
epicondyle

Trochlea

Capitulum

Head of
radius

Radial notch
of ulna

Coronoid
process of
ulna

FIGURE **8.8b** RIGHT ELBOW JOINT, ANTERIOR VIEW

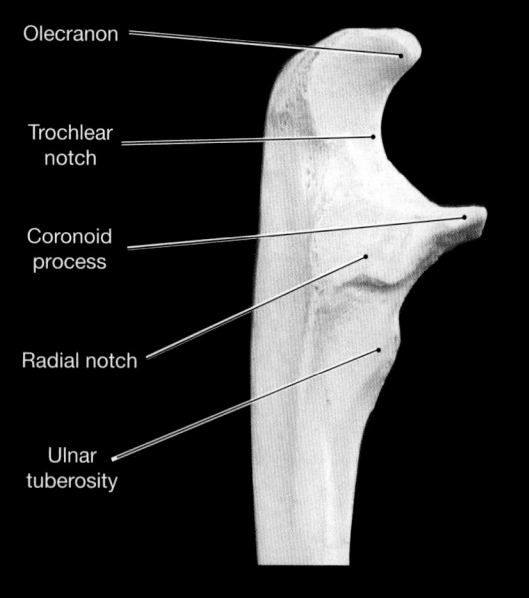

Olecranon

Trochlear
notch

Coronoid
process

Radial notch

Ulnar
tuberosity

FIGURE **8.8c** RIGHT ULNA, PROXIMAL, LATERAL VIEW

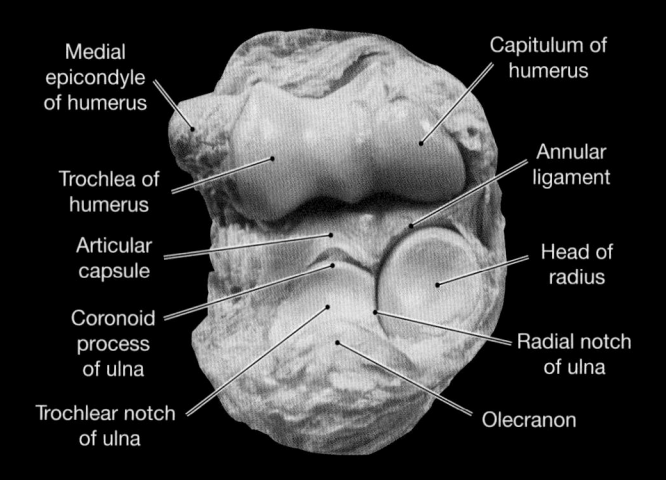

Medial
epicondyle
of humerus

Capitulum of
humerus

Annular
ligament

Trochlea of
humerus

Head of
radius

Articular
capsule

Coronoid
process
of ulna

Radial notch
of ulna

Trochlear notch
of ulna

Olecranon

FIGURE **8.8d** RIGHT ELBOW JOINT, ARTICULAR SURFACES

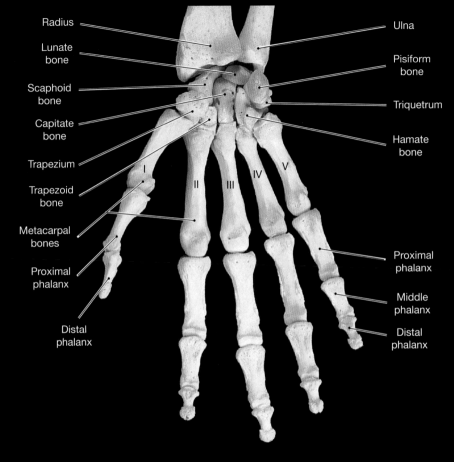

Radius
Lunate bone
Scaphoid bone
Capitate bone
Trapezium
Trapezoid bone
Metacarpal bones
Proximal phalanx
Distal phalanx

Ulna
Pisiform bone
Triquetrum
Hamate bone
Proximal phalanx
Middle phalanx
Distal phalanx

I II III IV V

FIGURE **8.10a** RIGHT HAND, ANTERIOR (PALMAR) VIEW

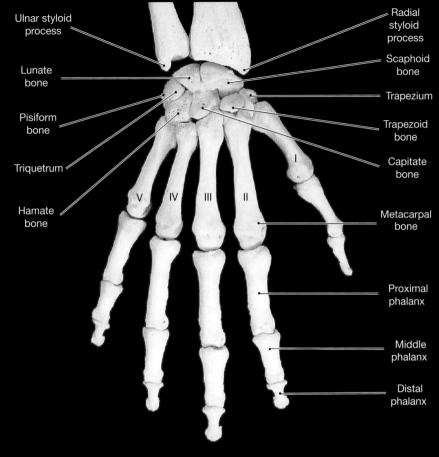

Ulnar styloid process
Lunate bone
Pisiform bone
Triquetrum
Hamate bone

Radial styloid process
Scaphoid bone
Trapezium
Trapezoid bone
Capitate bone
Metacarpal bone
Proximal phalanx
Middle phalanx
Distal phalanx

V IV III II I

FIGURE **8.10b** RIGHT HAND, POSTERIOR (DORSAL) VIEW

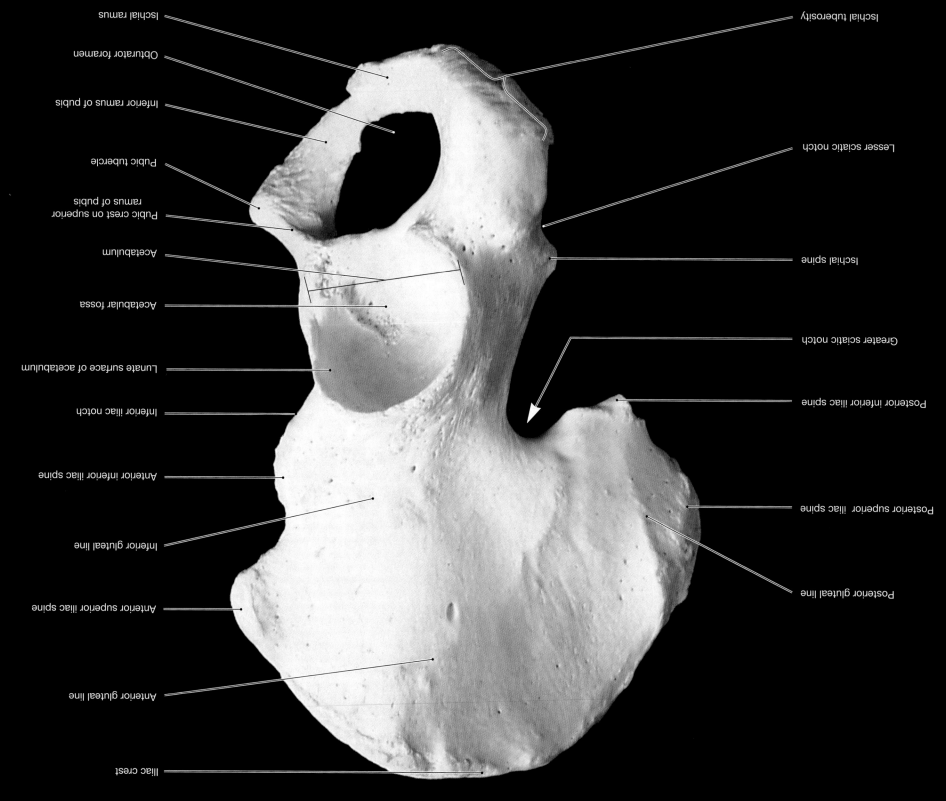

Ischial ramus

Obturator foramen

Inferior ramus of pubis

Pubic tubercle

Superior ramus of pubis

Pubic crest on superior ramus of pubis

Acetabulum

Acetabular fossa

Lunate surface of acetabulum

Inferior iliac notch

Anterior inferior iliac spine

Inferior gluteal line

Anterior superior iliac spine

Anterior gluteal line

Iliac crest

Ischial tuberosity

Lesser sciatic notch

Ischial spine

Greater sciatic notch

Posterior inferior iliac spine

Posterior superior iliac spine

Posterior gluteal line

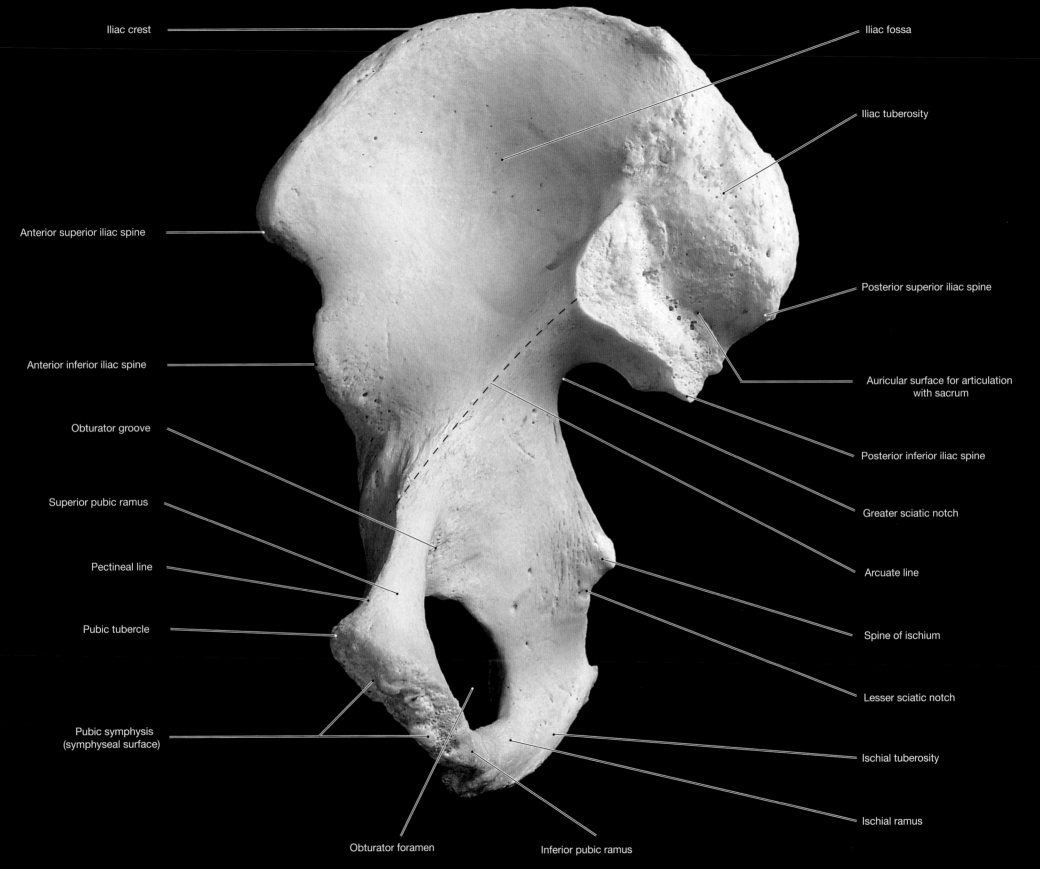

Iliac crest

Iliac fossa

Iliac tuberosity

Anterior superior iliac spine

Posterior superior iliac spine

Anterior inferior iliac spine

Auricular surface for articulation with sacrum

Obturator groove

Posterior inferior iliac spine

Superior pubic ramus

Greater sciatic notch

Pectineal line

Arcuate line

Pubic tubercle

Spine of ischium

Lesser sciatic notch

Pubic symphysis (symphyseal surface)

Ischial tuberosity

Ischial ramus

Obturator foramen

Inferior pubic ramus

FIGURE **9.1b** PELVIC GIRDLE, MEDIAL VIEW

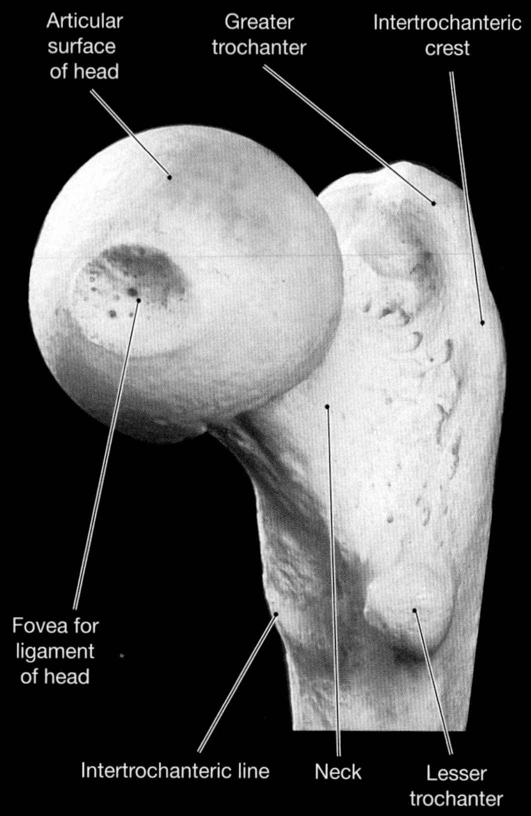

Articular
surface
of head

Greater
trochanter

Intertrochanteric
crest

Greater
trochanter

Intertrochanteric line

Neck

Articular
surface
of head

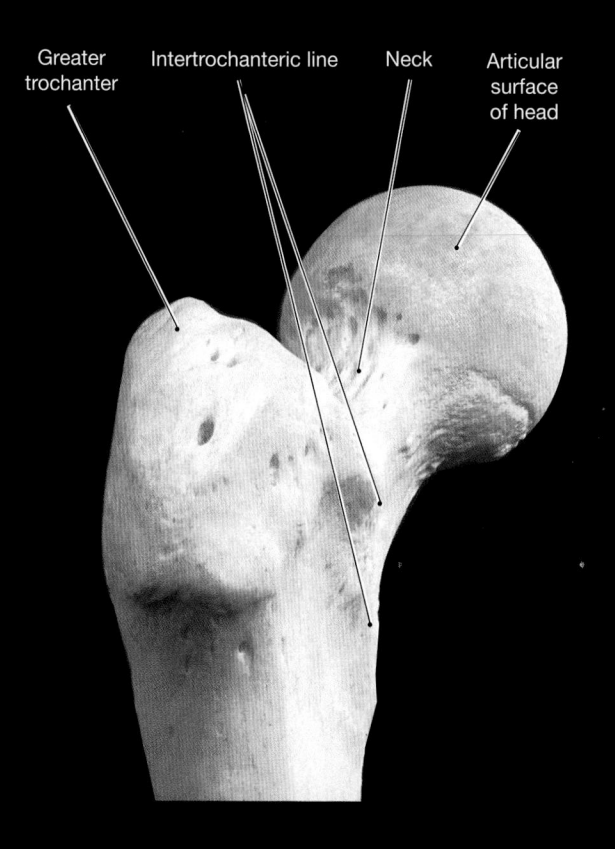

Fovea for
ligament
of head

**FIGURE 9.2a RIGHT
FEMUR, PROXIMAL,
MEDIAL VIEW**

Intertrochanteric line

Neck

Lesser
trochanter

**FIGURE 9.2b RIGHT
FEMUR, PROXIMAL,
LATERAL VIEW**

**FIGURE 9.3a RIGHT
FEMUR, SUPERIOR VIEW**

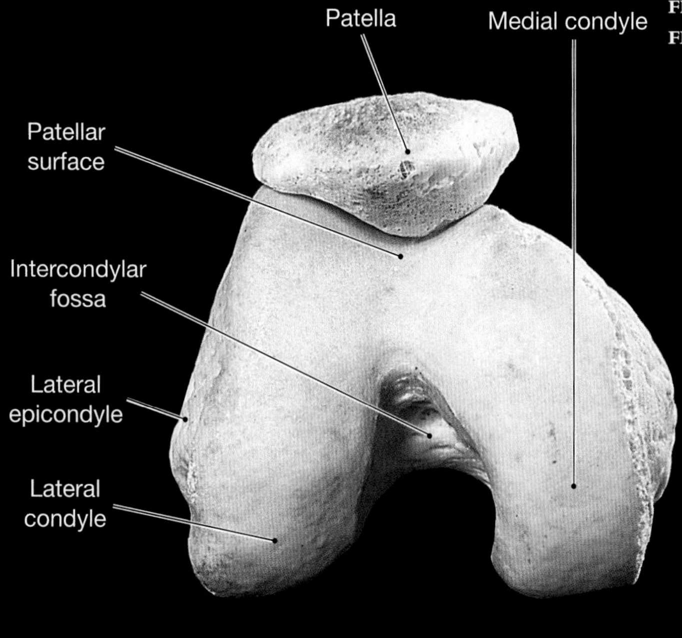

Neck

Greater
trochanter

Patella

Medial condyle

**FIGURE 9.3b RIGHT
FEMUR, INFERIOR VIEW**

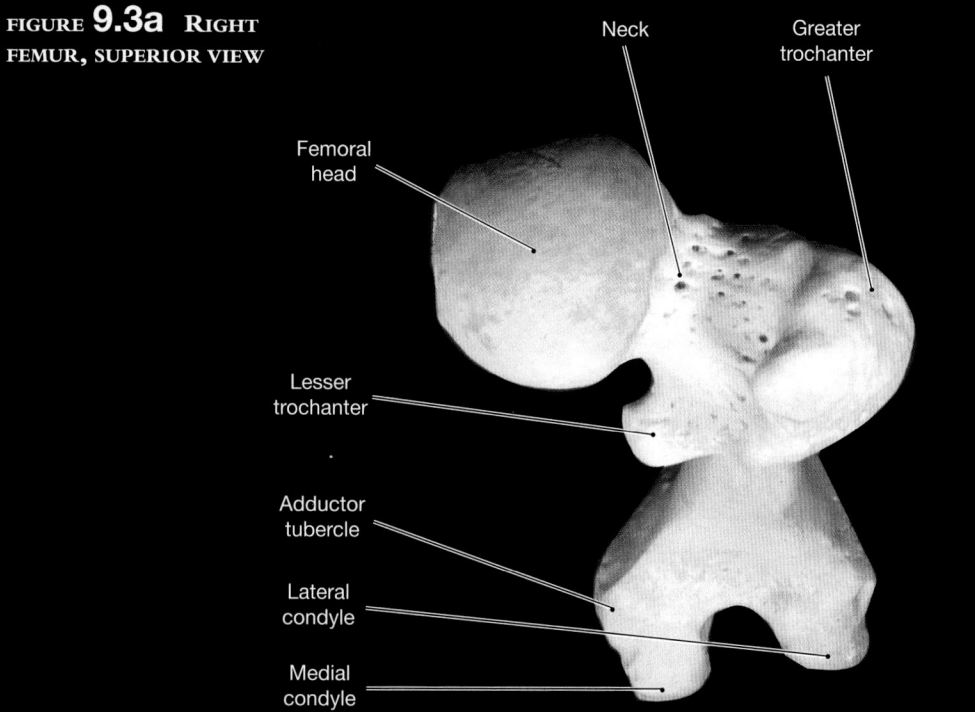

Femoral
head

Lesser
trochanter

Adductor
tubercle

Lateral
condyle

Medial
condyle

Patellar
surface

Intercondylar
fossa

Lateral
epicondyle

Lateral
condyle

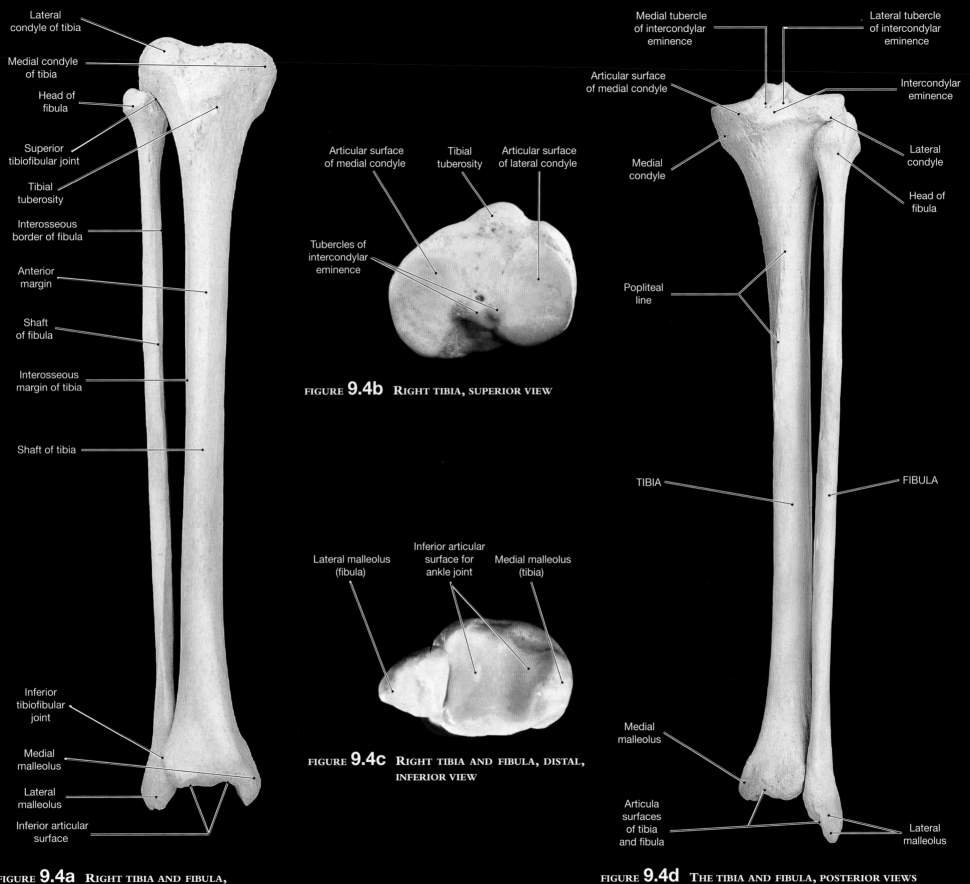

Lateral condyle of tibia

Medial condyle of tibia

Head of fibula

Superior tibiofibular joint

Tibial tuberosity

Interosseous border of fibula

Anterior margin

Shaft of fibula

Interosseous margin of tibia

Shaft of tibia

Inferior tibiofibular joint

Medial malleolus

Lateral malleolus

Inferior articular surface

FIGURE **9.4a** RIGHT TIBIA AND FIBULA, ANTERIOR VIEWS

Articular surface of medial condyle

Tibial tuberosity

Articular surface of lateral condyle

Tubercles of intercondylar eminence

FIGURE **9.4b** RIGHT TIBIA, SUPERIOR VIEW

Lateral malleolus (fibula)

Inferior articular surface for ankle joint

Medial malleolus (tibia)

FIGURE **9.4c** RIGHT TIBIA AND FIBULA, DISTAL, INFERIOR VIEW

Medial tubercle of intercondylar eminence

Lateral tubercle of intercondylar eminence

Articular surface of medial condyle

Intercondylar eminence

Medial condyle

Lateral condyle

Head of fibula

Popliteal line

TIBIA

FIBULA

Medial malleolus

Articula surfaces of tibia and fibula

Lateral malleolus

FIGURE **9.4d** THE TIBIA AND FIBULA, POSTERIOR VIEWS

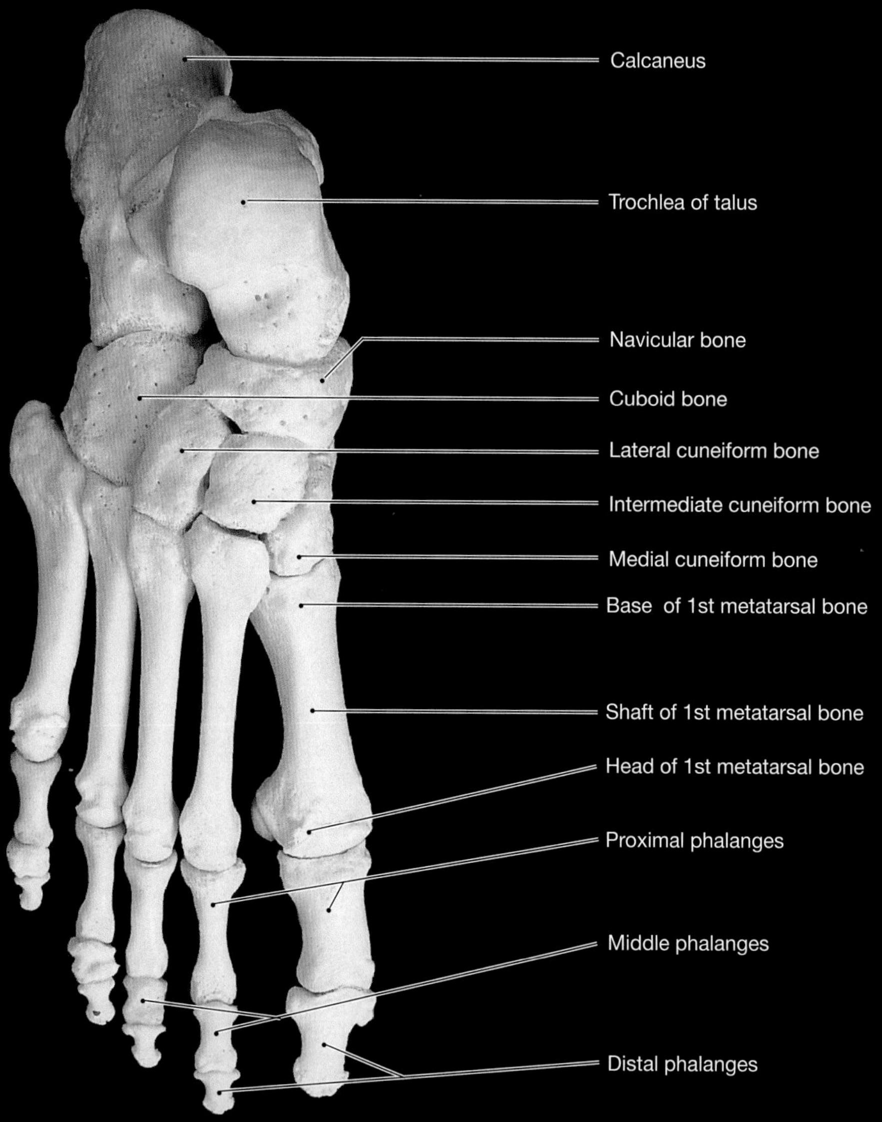

FIGURE **9.5a** RIGHT FOOT, SUPERIOR (DORSAL) VIEW

Distal phalanges

Middle phalanges

Proximal phalanges

Head of 1st metatarsal bone

Shaft of 1st metatarsal bone

Base of 1st metatarsal bone

Medial cuneiform bone

Intermediate cuneiform bone

Lateral cuneiform bone

Cuboid bone

Navicular bone

Trochlea of talus

Calcaneus

FIGURE **9.5b** RIGHT FOOT, INFERIOR (PLANTAR) VIEW

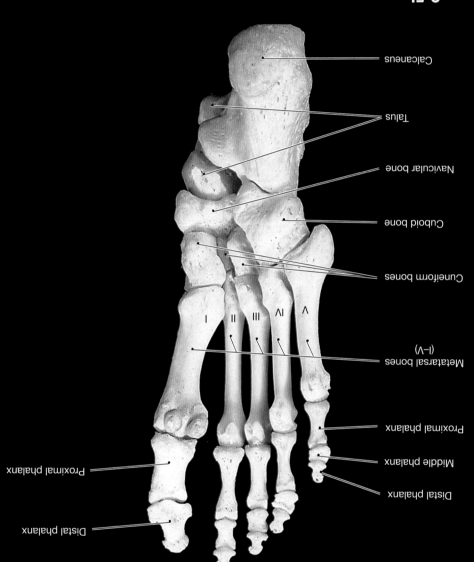

Calcaneus

Talus

Navicular bone

Cuboid bone

Cuneiform bones

Metatarsal bones (I–V)

Proximal phalanx

Middle phalanx

Distal phalanx

Proximal phalanx

Distal phalanx

I II III IV V

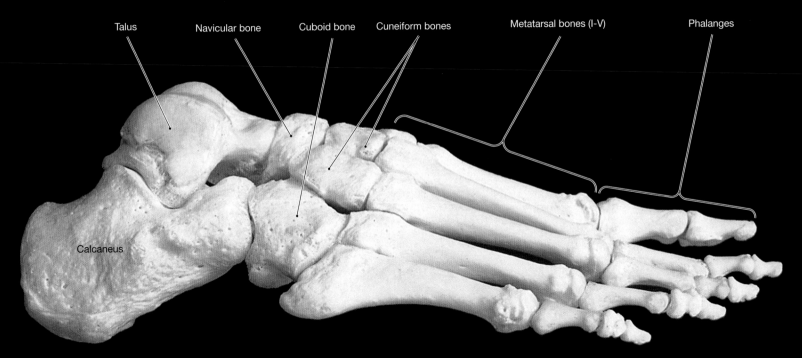

Talus   Navicular bone   Cuboid bone   Cuneiform bones   Metatarsal bones (I-V)   Phalanges

Calcaneus

FIGURE **9.5c** RIGHT FOOT, LATERAL VIEW

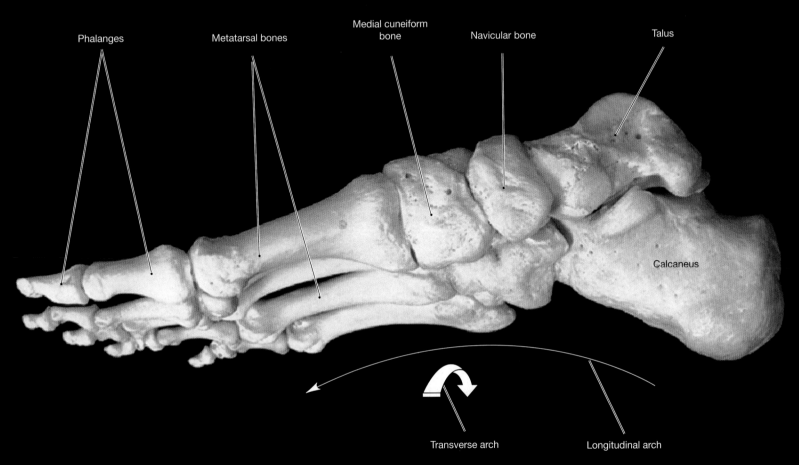

Phalanges   Metatarsal bones   Medial cuneiform bone   Navicular bone   Talus

Calcaneus

Transverse arch   Longitudinal arch

FIGURE **9.5d** RIGHT FOOT, MEDIAL VIEW

CADAVER IMAGES

FIGURE **1.1**   SUPERFICIAL DISSECTION OF THE FACE, LATERAL VIEW . C-2

FIGURE **1.2**   DEEP DISSECTION OF THE NECK, LATERAL VIEW C-2

FIGURE **1.3**   SURFACE ANATOMY OF THE ANTERIOR NECK C-3

FIGURE **1.4**   DISSECTION OF THE ANTERIOR NECK C-3

FIGURE **1.5**   SHOULDER AND NECK, ANTERIOR VIEW C-3

FIGURE **2.1**   THE HEAD IN HORIZONTAL SECTION C-4

FIGURE **2.2**   THE HEAD IN SAGITTAL SECTION C-5

FIGURE **3.1**   TRUNK, ANTERIOR VIEW C-6

FIGURE **3.2**   TRUNK, POSTERIOR VIEW C-7

FIGURE **4.1**   THE HEART AND LUNGS, ANTERIOR VIEW C-8

FIGURE **4.2a**   RIGHT LUNG, MEDIAL VIEW C-8

FIGURE **4.2b**   LEFT LUNG, MEDIAL VIEW C-8

FIGURE **4.3a**   PAINTED SEGMENTS OF THE RIGHT LUNG,
ANTERIOR VIEW C-9

FIGURE **4.3b**   PAINTED SEGMENTS OF THE LEFT LUNG,
ANTERIOR VIEW C-9

FIGURE **5.1**   ABDOMINAL WALL, ANTERIOR VIEW C-9

FIGURE **5.2**   ABDOMINAL MUSCLES C-10

FIGURE **5.3a**   ABDOMINAL DISSECTION, SUPERIOR PORTION, ANTERIOR
VIEW C-10

FIGURE **5.3b**   ABDOMINAL DISSECTION, INFERIOR PORTION,
ANTERIOR VIEW C-11

FIGURE **5.3c**   ABDOMINAL DISSECTION, GREATER OMENTUM
REFLECTED C-11

FIGURE **5.3d**   ABDOMINAL DISSECTION, DUODENAL REGION C-12

FIGURE **5.3e**   APPENDIX IN SITU C-12

FIGURE **5.4a**   LIVER AND GALLBLADDER, SUPERIOR VIEW C-13

FIGURE **5.4b**   LIVER AND GALLBLADDER, INFERIOR VIEW C-13

FIGURE **5.4c**   LIVER AND GALLBLADDER IN SITU C-14

FIGURE **5.4d**   CORROSION CAST OF LIVER C-14

FIGURE **5.5**   NORMAL AND ABNORMAL COLONOSCOPE C-15

FIGURE **5.6a**   SPLEEN, ANTERIOR VIEW C-15

FIGURE **5.6b**   CAST OF SPLENIC AND PANCREATIC VESSELS C-15

FIGURE **5.7a**   SUPERIOR MESENTERIC ARTERY C-16

FIGURE **5.7b**   INFERIOR MESENTERIC VESSELS C-16

FIGURE **5.8a**   ABDOMINAL CAVITY, HORIZONTAL SECTION AT T_{12} . . . C-17

FIGURE **5.8b**   ABDOMINAL CAVITY, HORIZONTAL SECTION AT L_1 . . . . C-18

FIGURE **5.9**   THE KIDNEYS AND ASSOCIATED STRUCTURES C-19

FIGURE **5.10a**   THE INFERIOR PELVIS, SUPERIOR VIEW C-20

FIGURE **5.10b**   VESSELS OF INFERIOR PELVIS, MEDIAL VIEW C-21

FIGURE **6.1**   RIGHT LOWER QUADRANT, MALE C-21

FIGURE **6.2**   RIGHT HIP, SUPERFICIAL DISSECTION, POSTERIOR VIEW . C-22

FIGURE **6.3**   RIGHT HIP AND THIGH, ANTERIOR VIEW C-22

FIGURE **6.4a**   RIGHT FOOT, SUPERFICIAL DISSECTION, LATERAL VIEW . C-23

FIGURE **6.4b**   RIGHT FOOT, INTRINSIC MUSCLES (SUPERFICIAL),
PLANTAR VIEW C-23

FIGURE **6.5a**   MODEL OF THE RIGHT HAND, POSTERIOR VIEW C-24

FIGURE **6.5b**   MODEL OF THE ELBOW JOINT, LONGITUDINAL SECTION . C-24

FIGURE **6.5c**   MODEL OF THE KNEE JOINT, SAGITTAL SECTION C-24

FIGURE 1.1 SUPERFICIAL DISSECTION OF THE FACE, LATERAL VIEW

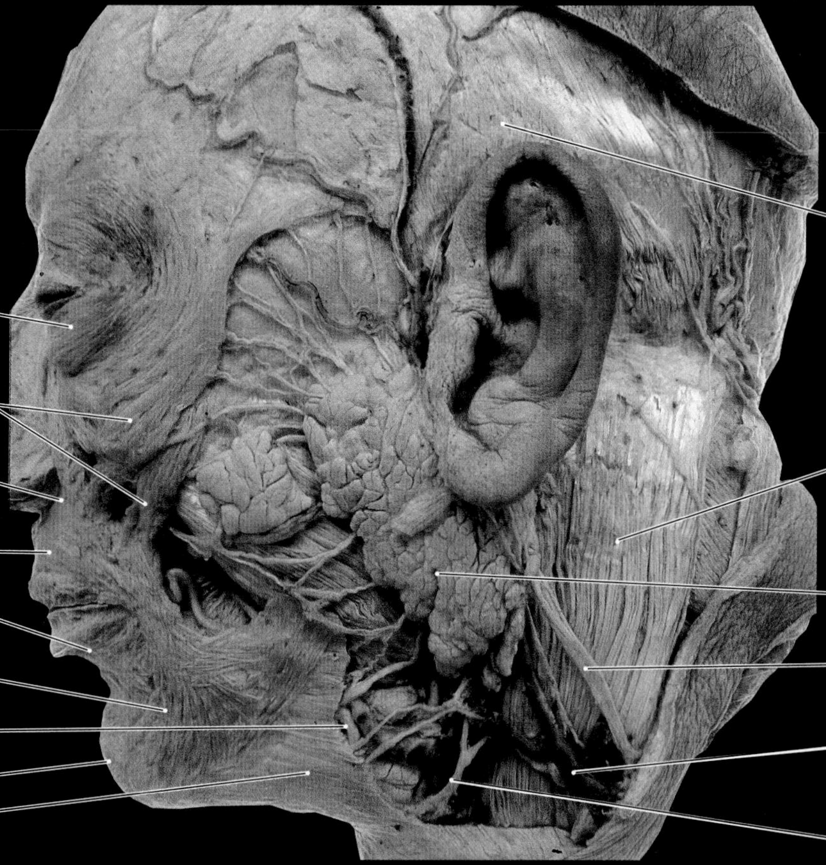

Temporoparietalis muscle

Orbicularis oculi muscle

Zygomaticus muscle (minor and major)

Levator labii superioris muscle

Orbicularis oris muscle

Sternocleidomastoid muscle

Depressor labii inferioris muscle

Parotid salivary gland

Depressor anguli oris muscle

Great auricular nerve

Facial artery

External jugular vein

Mentalis muscle

Platysma

Transverse cervical nerve

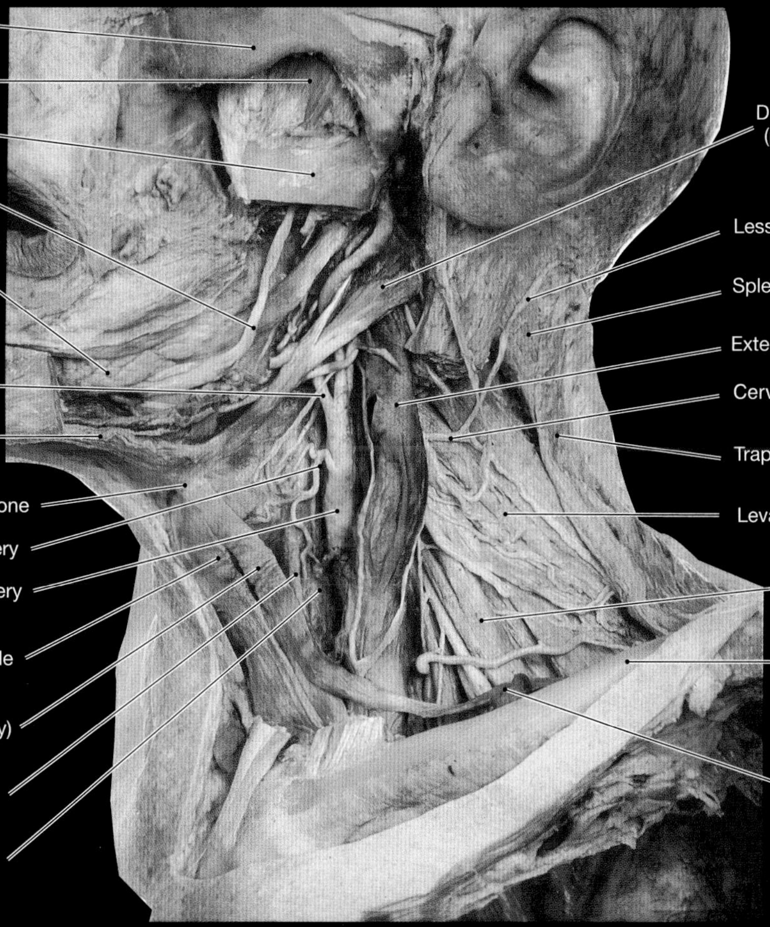

Zygomatic arch

Temporalis muscle

Mandible (cut)

Lingual nerve

Digastric muscle (posterior belly)

Lesser occipital nerve

Sublingual salivary gland

Splenius capitis muscle

External jugular vein

Common carotid artery

Cervical nerves

Digastric muscle (anterior belly)

Trapezius muscle

Hyoid bone

Levator scapulae muscle

Superior thyroid artery

Common carotid artery

Medial scalene muscle

Sternohyoid muscle

Omohyoid muscle (superior belly)

Clavicle

Sternothyroid muscle

Omohyoid muscle (superior belly)

Thyroid gland

FIGURE 1.2 DEEP DISSECTION OF THE NECK, LATERAL VIEW

FIGURE 1.3 **SURFACE**
ANATOMY OF THE
ANTERIOR NECK

Platysma

Thyroid cartilage
of the larynx

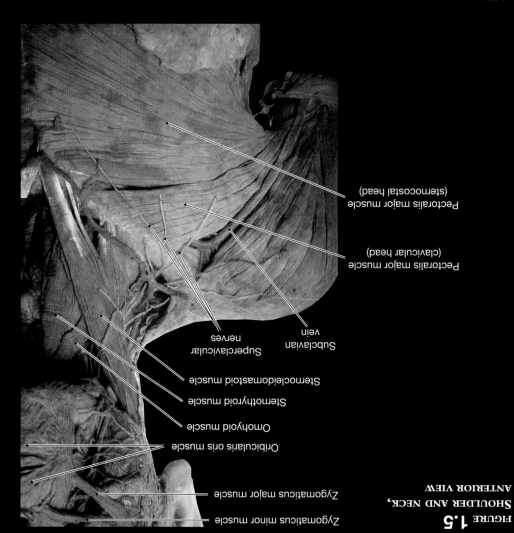

FIGURE 1.5
SHOULDER AND NECK,
ANTERIOR VIEW

Pectoralis major muscle
(sternocostal head)

Pectoralis major muscle
(clavicular head)

Subclavian
vein

Supraclavicular
nerves

Sternocleidomastoid muscle

Sternothyroid muscle

Omohyoid muscle

Orbicularis oris muscle

Zygomaticus major muscle

Zygomaticus minor muscle

FIGURE 1.4
DISSECTION OF THE
ANTERIOR NECK

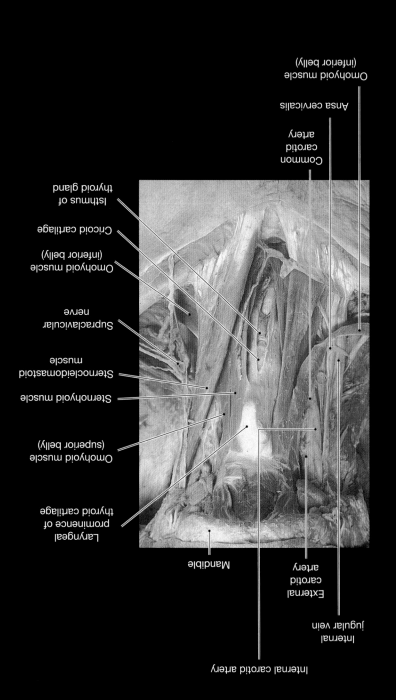

Mandible

Internal
jugular vein

External
carotid
artery

Internal carotid artery

Supraclavicular
nerve

Sternocleidomastoid
muscle

Sternohyoid muscle

Omohyoid muscle
(superior belly)

Laryngeal
prominence of
thyroid cartilage

Omohyoid muscle
(inferior belly)

Cricoid cartilage

Isthmus of
thyroid gland

Common
carotid
artery

Ansa cervicalis

Omohyoid muscle
(inferior belly)

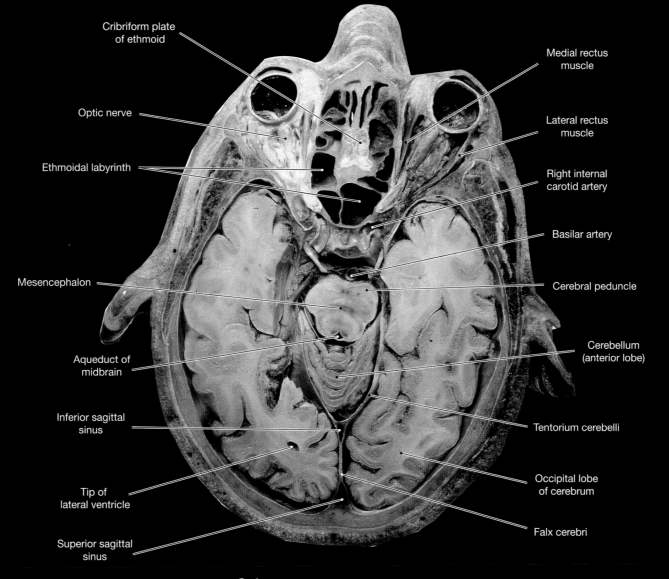

Cribriform plate
of ethmoid

Optic nerve

Ethmoidal labyrinth

Mesencephalon

Aqueduct of
midbrain

Inferior sagittal
sinus

Tip of
lateral ventricle

Superior sagittal
sinus

Medial rectus
muscle

Lateral rectus
muscle

Right internal
carotid artery

Basilar artery

Cerebral peduncle

Cerebellum
(anterior lobe)

Tentorium cerebelli

Occipital lobe
of cerebrum

Falx cerebri

FIGURE **2.1** THE HEAD IN HORIZONTAL SECTION

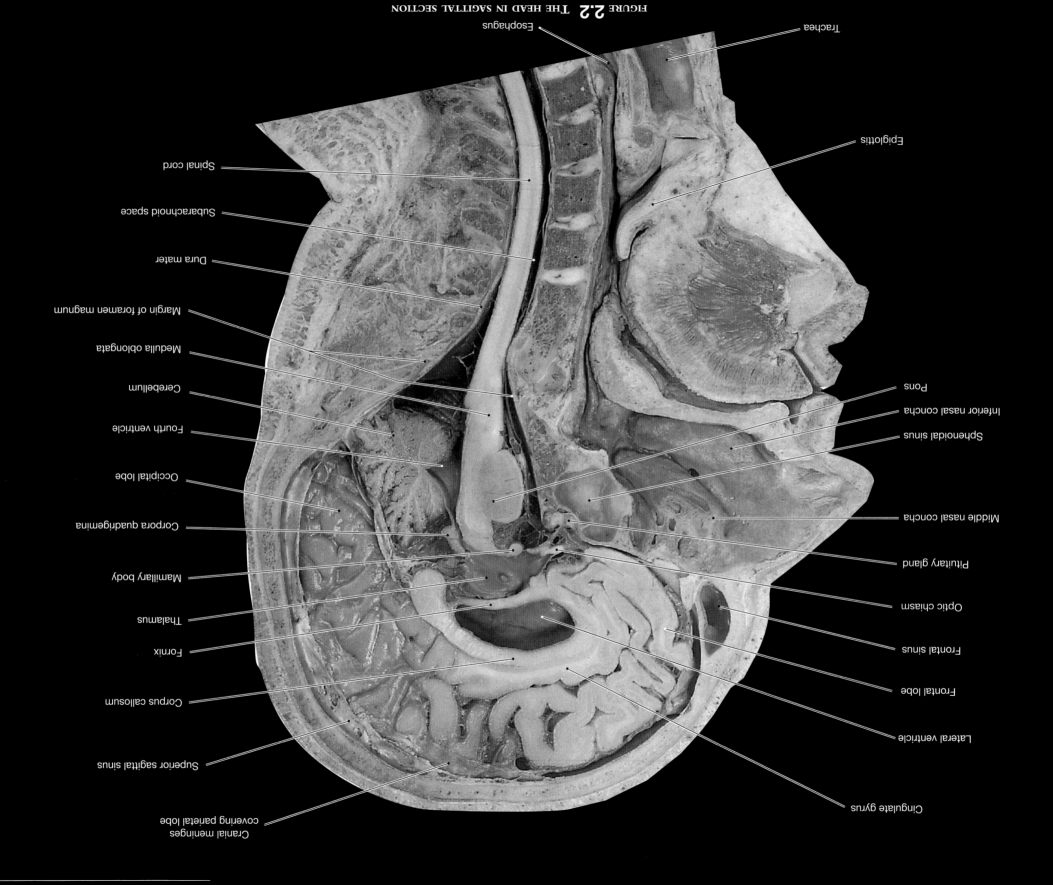

FIGURE 2.2 THE HEAD IN SAGITTAL SECTION

Esophagus

Trachea

Epiglottis

Spinal cord

Subarachnoid space

Dura mater

Margin of foramen magnum

Medulla oblongata

Pons

Inferior nasal concha

Cerebellum

Sphenoidal sinus

Fourth ventricle

Occipital lobe

Middle nasal concha

Corpora quadrigemina

Pituitary gland

Mamillary body

Optic chiasm

Thalamus

Frontal sinus

Fornix

Corpus callosum

Frontal lobe

Superior sagittal sinus

Lateral ventricle

Cranial meninges
covering parietal lobe

Cingulate gyrus

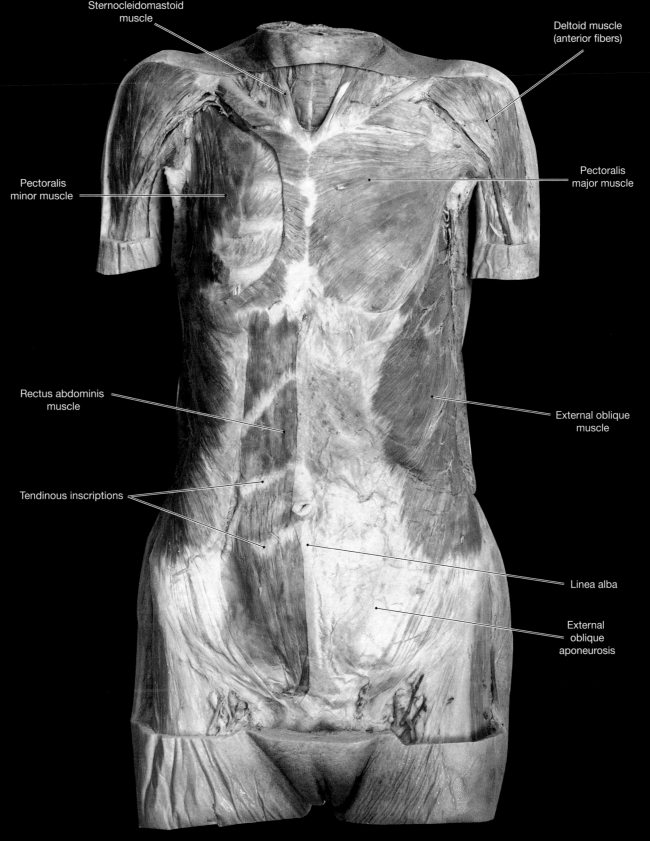

Sternocleidomastoid muscle

Deltoid muscle (anterior fibers)

Pectoralis minor muscle

Pectoralis major muscle

Rectus abdominis muscle

External oblique muscle

Tendinous inscriptions

Linea alba

External oblique aponeurosis

FIGURE **3.1** TRUNK, ANTERIOR VIEW

FIGURE 3.2 TRUNK, POSTERIOR VIEW

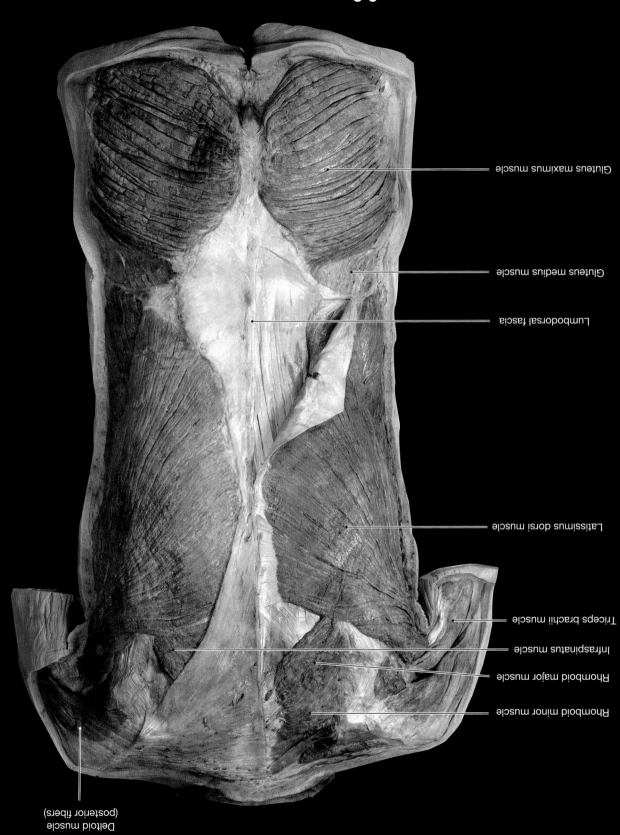

Gluteus maximus muscle

Gluteus medius muscle

Lumbodorsal fascia

Latissimus dorsi muscle

Triceps brachii muscle

Infraspinatus muscle

Rhomboid major muscle

Rhomboid minor muscle

Deltoid muscle
(posterior fibers)

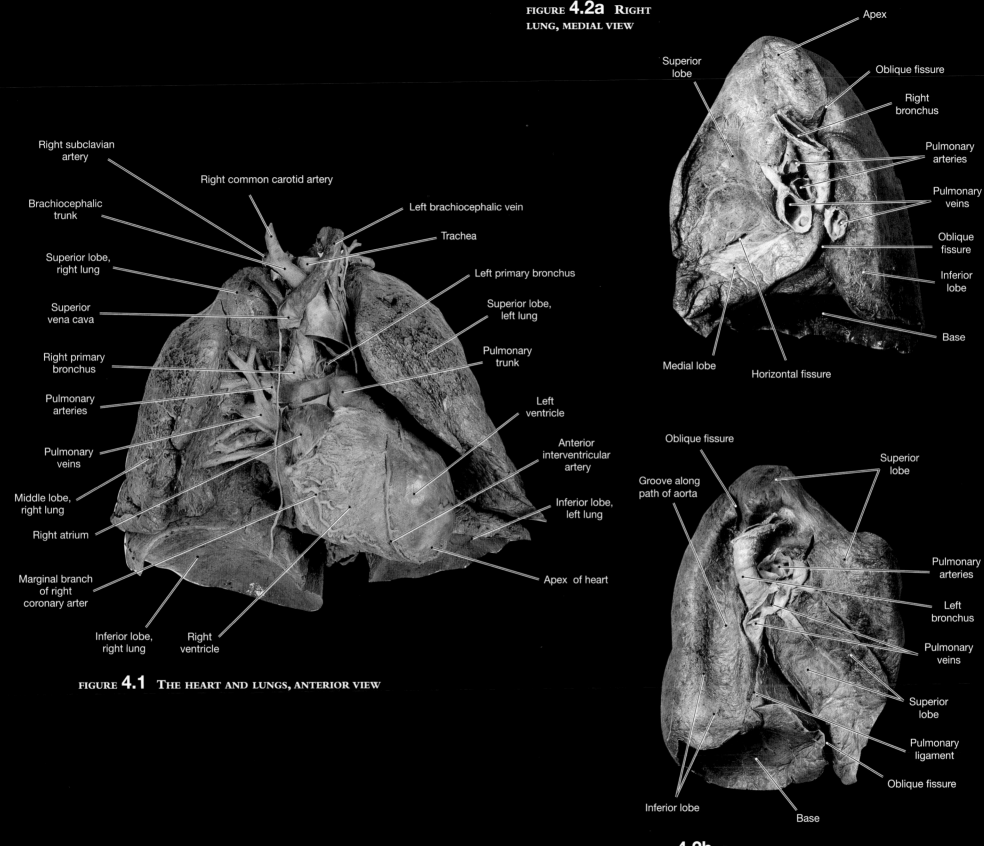

FIGURE **4.2a** RIGHT LUNG, MEDIAL VIEW

Apex

Superior lobe

Oblique fissure

Right bronchus

Pulmonary arteries

Pulmonary veins

Oblique fissure

Inferior lobe

Base

Medial lobe

Horizontal fissure

Right subclavian artery

Right common carotid artery

Brachiocephalic trunk

Left brachiocephalic vein

Trachea

Superior lobe, right lung

Left primary bronchus

Superior vena cava

Superior lobe, left lung

Right primary bronchus

Pulmonary trunk

Pulmonary arteries

Left ventricle

Pulmonary veins

Anterior interventricular artery

Middle lobe, right lung

Inferior lobe, left lung

Right atrium

Marginal branch of right coronary arter

Apex of heart

Inferior lobe, right lung

Right ventricle

FIGURE **4.1** THE HEART AND LUNGS, ANTERIOR VIEW

Oblique fissure

Superior lobe

Groove along path of aorta

Pulmonary arteries

Left bronchus

Pulmonary veins

Superior lobe

Pulmonary ligament

Oblique fissure

Inferior lobe

Base

FIGURE **4.2b** LEFT LUNG, MEDIAL VIEW

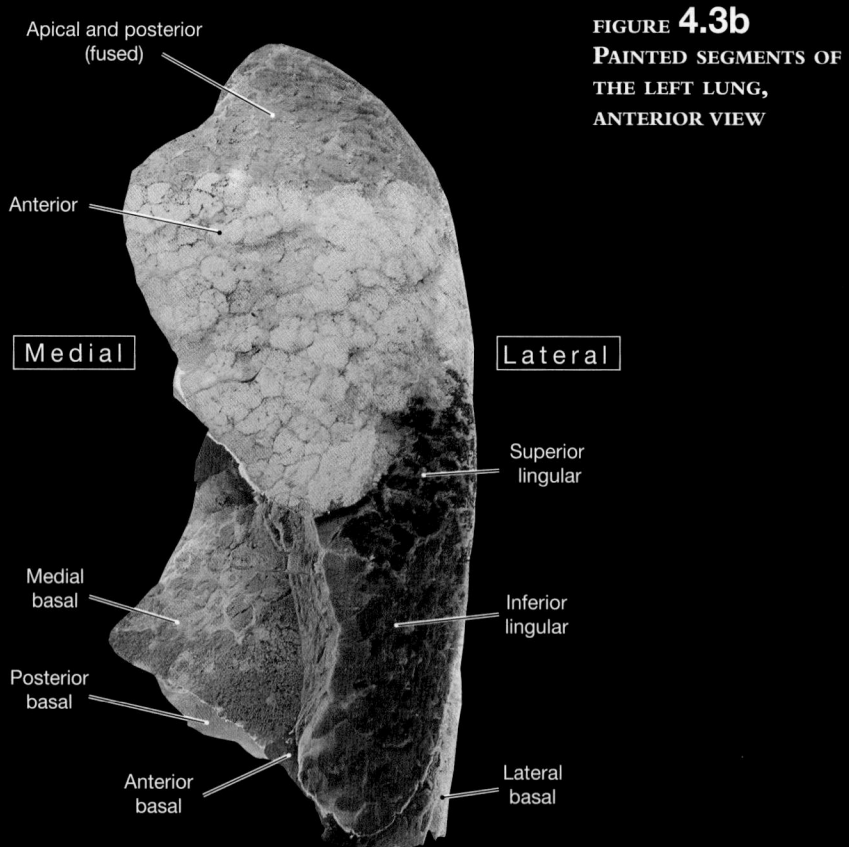

FIGURE 4.3a
PAINTED SEGMENTS OF THE RIGHT LUNG, ANTERIOR VIEW

Apical

Anterior

Lateral

Medial

Lateral
Medial

Anterior basal

Lateral basal

Medial basal

Posterior basal

FIGURE 4.3b
PAINTED SEGMENTS OF THE LEFT LUNG, ANTERIOR VIEW

Apical and posterior (fused)

Anterior

Medial

Lateral

Medial basal

Posterior basal

Anterior basal

Superior lingular

Inferior lingular

Lateral basal

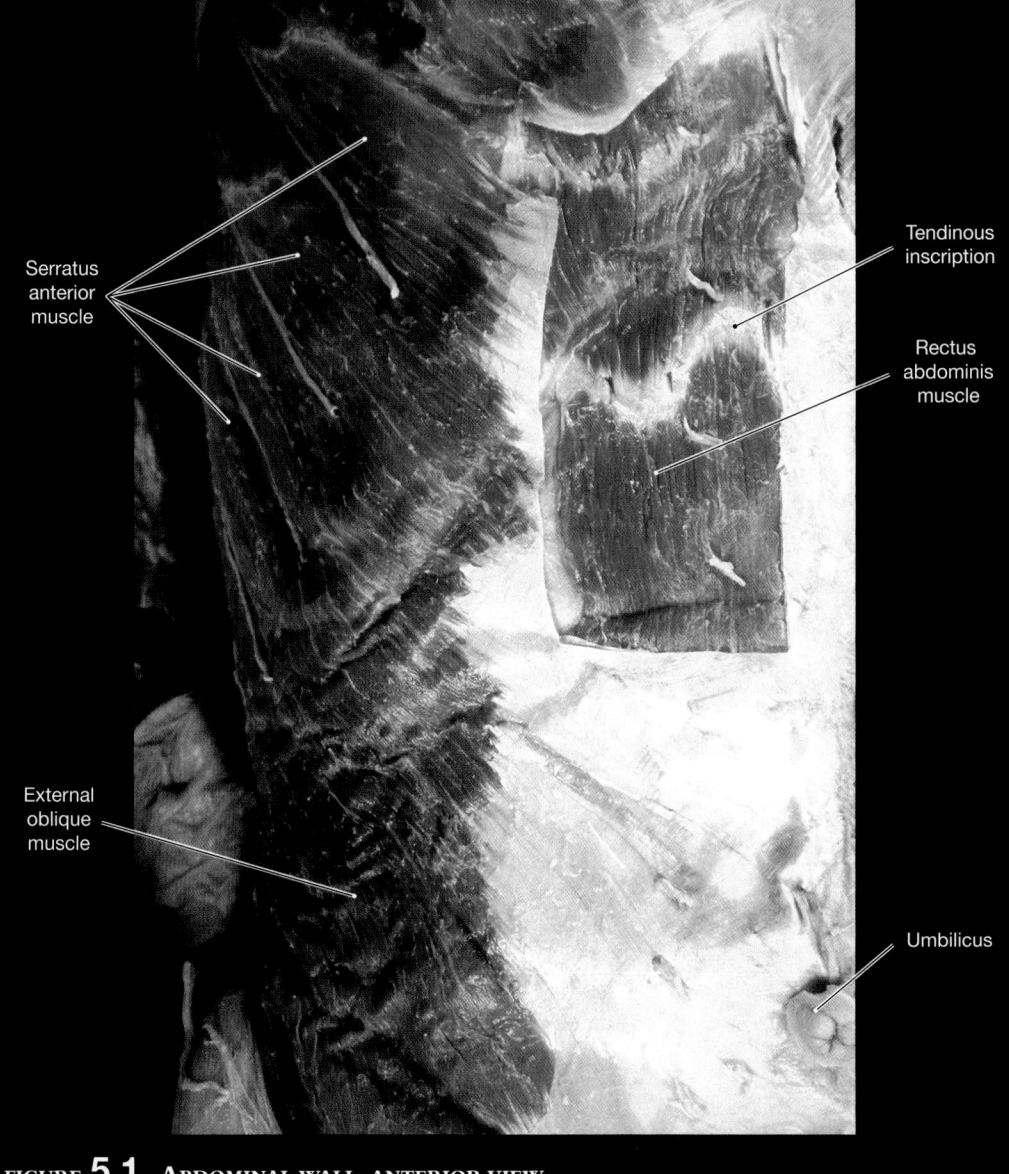

Serratus anterior muscle

External oblique muscle

Tendinous inscription

Rectus abdominis muscle

Umbilicus

FIGURE 5.1   ABDOMINAL WALL, ANTERIOR VIEW

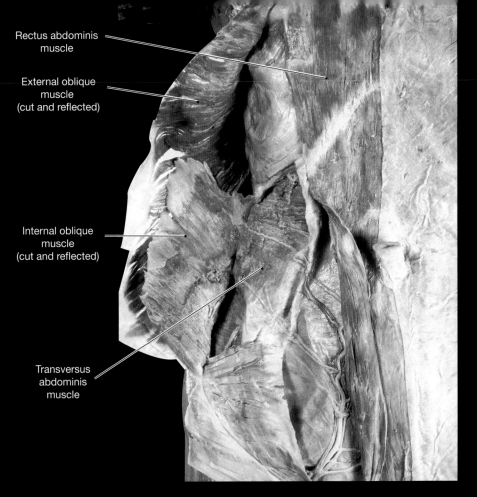

Rectus abdominis
muscle

External oblique
muscle
(cut and reflected)

Internal oblique
muscle
(cut and reflected)

Transversus
abdominis
muscle

FIGURE **5.2**
ABDOMINAL MUSCLES

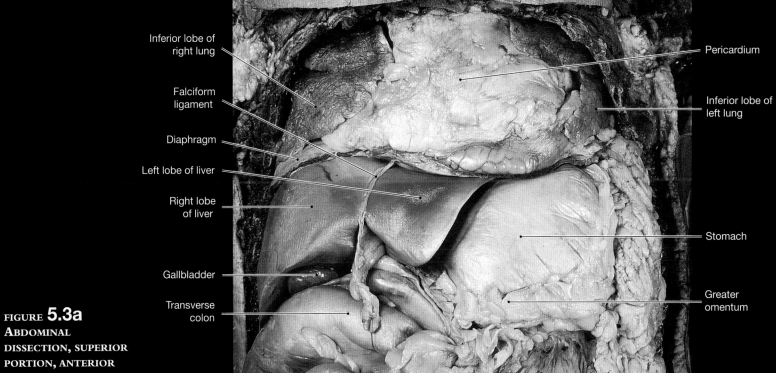

Inferior lobe of
right lung

Falciform
ligament

Diaphragm

Left lobe of liver

Right lobe
of liver

Gallbladder

Transverse
colon

Pericardium

Inferior lobe of
left lung

Stomach

Greater
omentum

FIGURE **5.3a**
ABDOMINAL
DISSECTION, SUPERIOR
PORTION, ANTERIOR

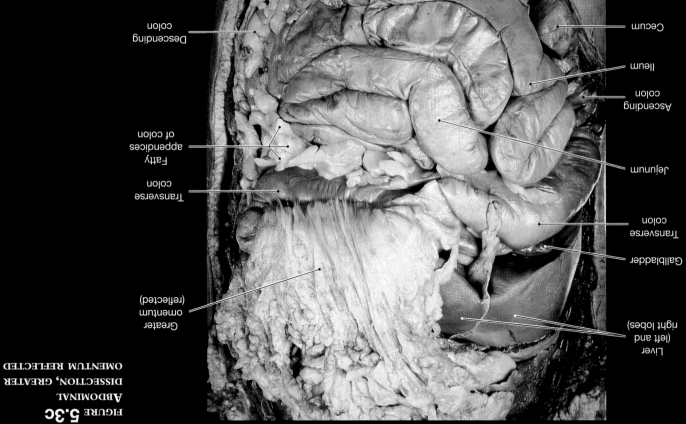

FIGURE 5.3C ABDOMINAL DISSECTION, GREATER OMENTUM REFLECTED

Descending colon

Cecum

Ileum

Ascending colon

Jejunum

Fatty appendices of colon

Transverse colon

Transverse colon

Gallbladder

Greater omentum (reflected)

Liver (left and right lobes)

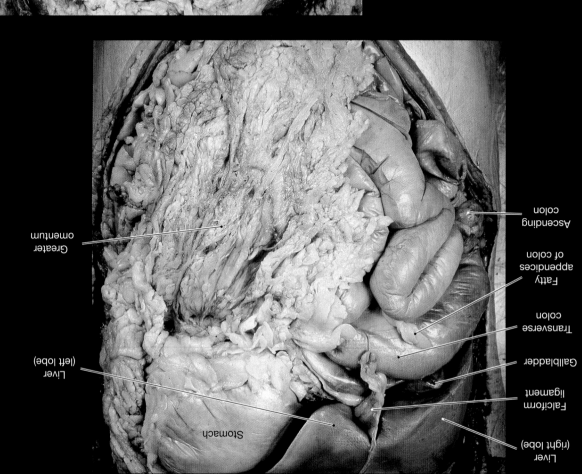

FIGURE 5.3b ABDOMINAL DISSECTION, INFERIOR PORTION, ANTERIOR VIEW

Greater omentum

Ascending colon

Fatty appendices of colon

Transverse colon

Gallbladder

Falciform ligament

Liver (right lobe)

Liver (left lobe)

Stomach

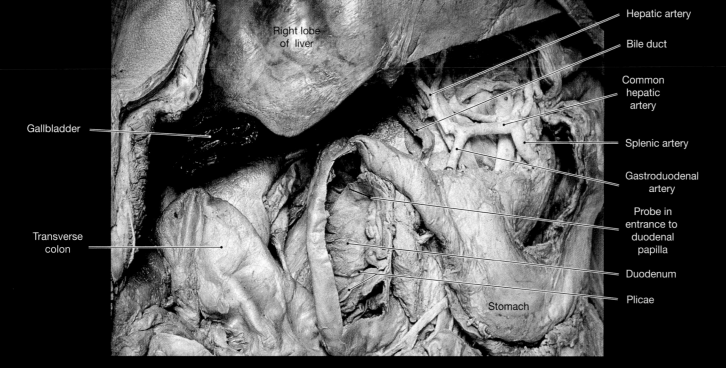

Right lobe of liver

Gallbladder

Transverse colon

Hepatic artery

Bile duct

Common hepatic artery

Splenic artery

Gastroduodenal artery

Probe in entrance to duodenal papilla

Duodenum

Plicae

Stomach

FIGURE **5.3d** ABDOMINAL DISSECTION, DUODENAL REGION

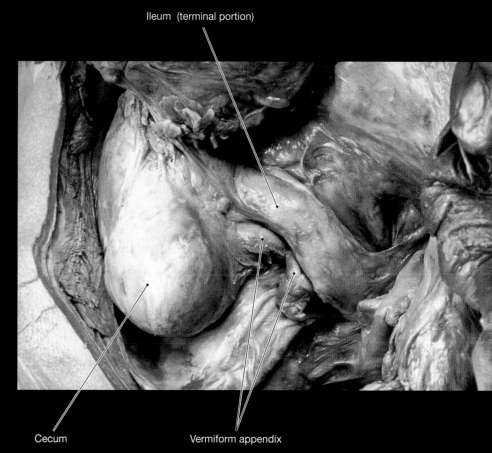

Ileum (terminal portion)

FIGURE **5.3e**
APPENDIX IN SITU

Cecum

Vermiform appendix

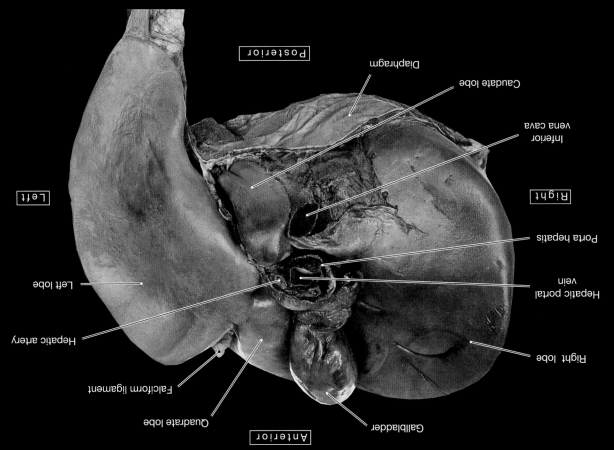

Posterior

Diaphragm

Caudate lobe

Inferior vena cava

Left

Right

Porta hepatis

Left lobe

Hepatic portal vein

Hepatic artery

Right lobe

Falciform ligament

Quadrate lobe

Gallbladder

Anterior

FIGURE 5.4b LIVER AND GALLBLADDER, INFERIOR VIEW

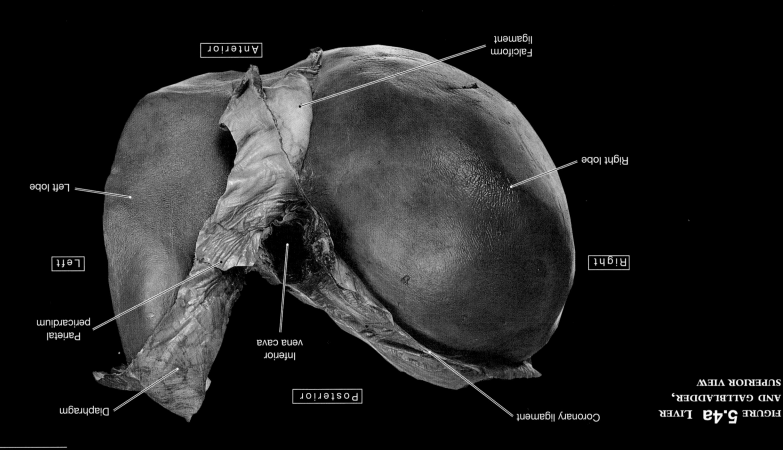

Anterior

Falciform ligament

Left lobe

Right lobe

Left

Right

Parietal pericardium

Inferior vena cava

Diaphragm

Coronary ligament

Posterior

FIGURE 5.4a LIVER AND GALLBLADDER, SUPERIOR VIEW

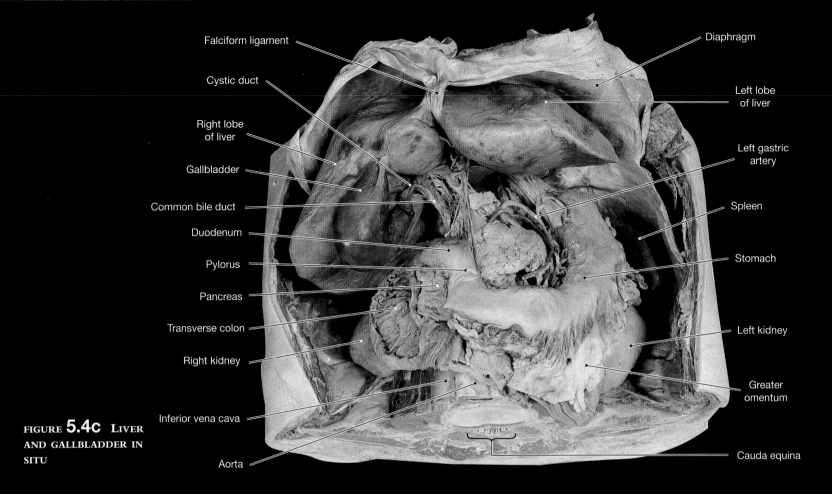

Falciform ligament

Cystic duct

Right lobe
of liver

Gallbladder

Common bile duct

Duodenum

Pylorus

Pancreas

Transverse colon

Right kidney

Inferior vena cava

Aorta

Diaphragm

Left lobe
of liver

Left gastric
artery

Spleen

Stomach

Left kidney

Greater
omentum

Cauda equina

FIGURE 5.4c LIVER AND GALLBLADDER IN SITU

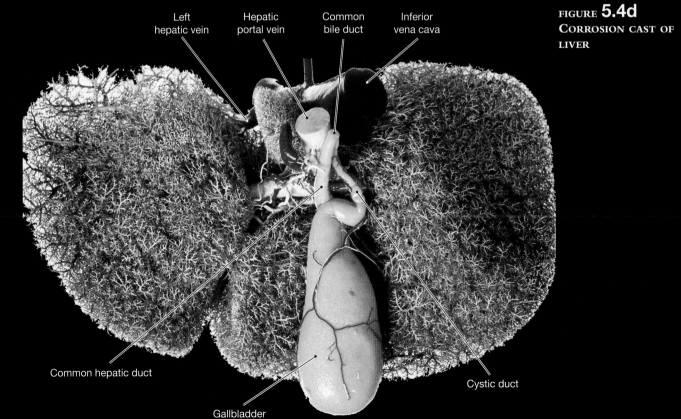

FIGURE 5.4d CORROSION CAST OF LIVER

Left
hepatic vein

Hepatic
portal vein

Common
bile duct

Inferior
vena cava

Common hepatic duct

Gallbladder

Cystic duct

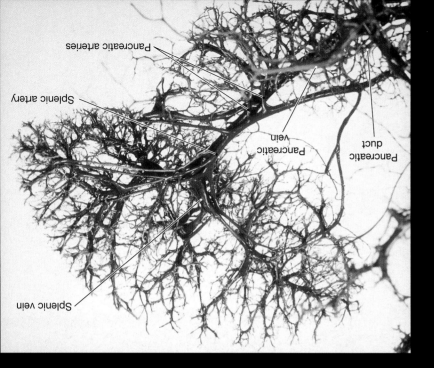

FIGURE 5.6b
CAST OF SPLENIC AND PANCREATIC VESSELS

Pancreatic arteries

Splenic artery

Pancreatic vein

Pancreatic duct

Splenic vein

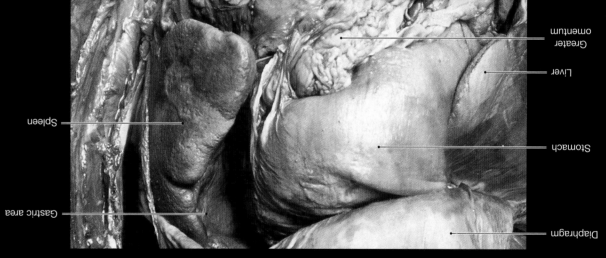

FIGURE 5.6a
SPLEEN, ANTERIOR VIEW

Greater omentum

Liver

Stomach

Diaphragm

Spleen

Gastric area

FIGURE 5.5
NORMAL AND ABNORMAL COLONOSCOPE

Normal section of colon, demonstrating region of previous polyp removal.

Polyp on wall of colon

FIGURE **5.7a**
SUPERIOR MESENTERIC
ARTERY

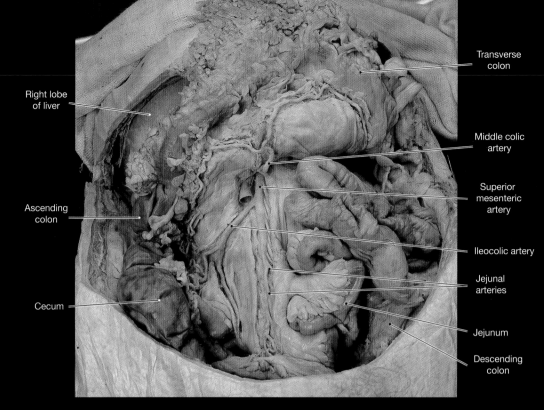

Transverse
colon

Right lobe
of liver

Middle colic
artery

Superior
mesenteric
artery

Ascending
colon

Ileocolic artery

Jejunal
arteries

Cecum

Jejunum

Descending
colon

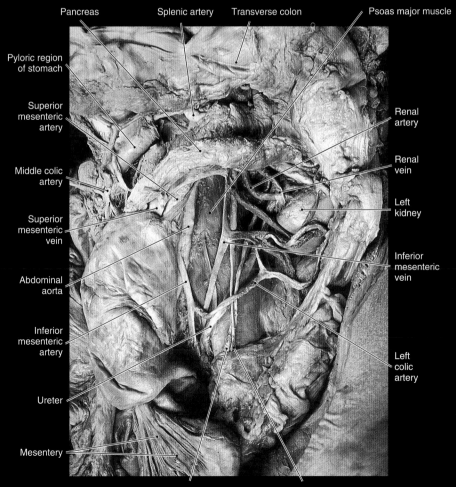

Pancreas   Splenic artery   Transverse colon   Psoas major muscle

Pyloric region
of stomach

Superior
mesenteric
artery

Renal
artery

Renal
vein

Middle colic
artery

Superior
mesenteric
vein

Left
kidney

Abdominal
aorta

Inferior
mesenteric
vein

Inferior
mesenteric
artery

Left
colic
artery

Ureter

Mesentery

Gonadal artery   Gonadal vein

FIGURE **5.7b**
INFERIOR MESENTERIC
VESSELS

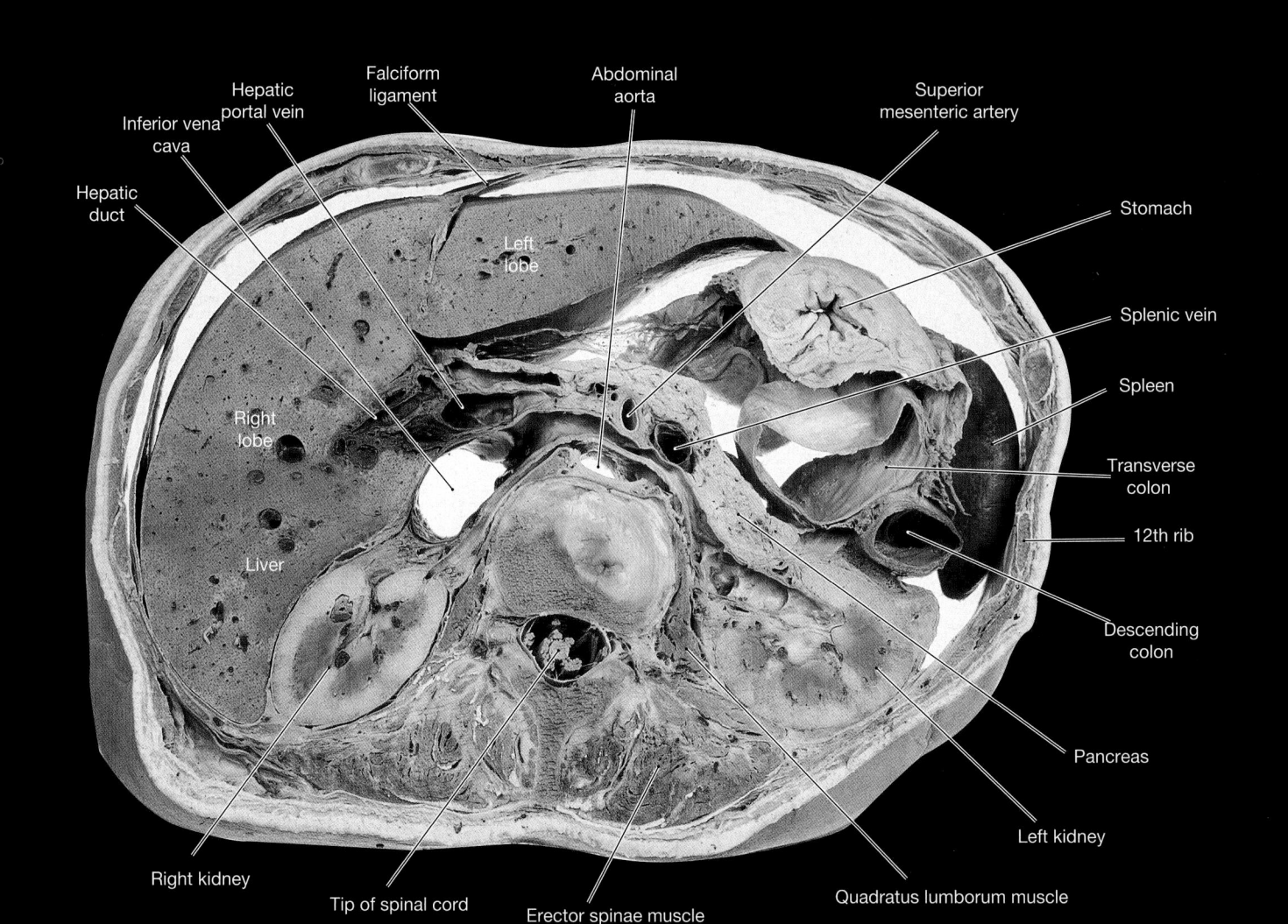

Hepatic portal vein

Inferior vena cava

Falciform ligament

Abdominal aorta

Superior mesenteric artery

Hepatic duct

Stomach

Left lobe

Splenic vein

Spleen

Right lobe

Transverse colon

12th rib

Liver

Descending colon

Pancreas

Left kidney

Right kidney

Tip of spinal cord

Erector spinae muscle

Quadratus lumborum muscle

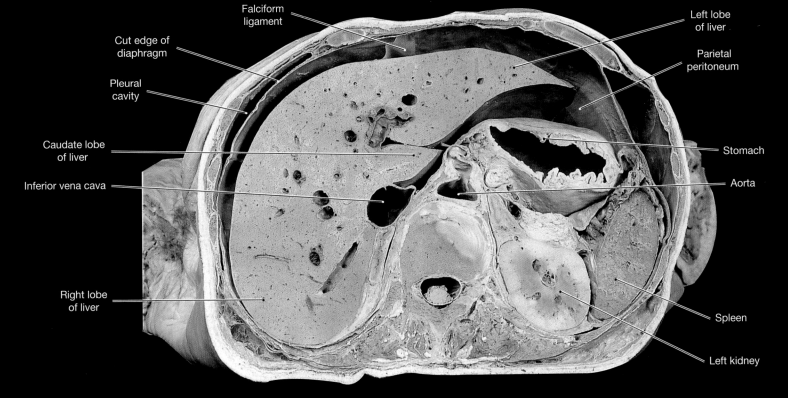

Falciform ligament

Cut edge of diaphragm

Pleural cavity

Caudate lobe of liver

Inferior vena cava

Right lobe of liver

Left lobe of liver

Parietal peritoneum

Stomach

Aorta

Spleen

Left kidney

FIGURE **5.8b** ABDOMINAL CAVITY, HORIZONTAL SECTION AT L_1

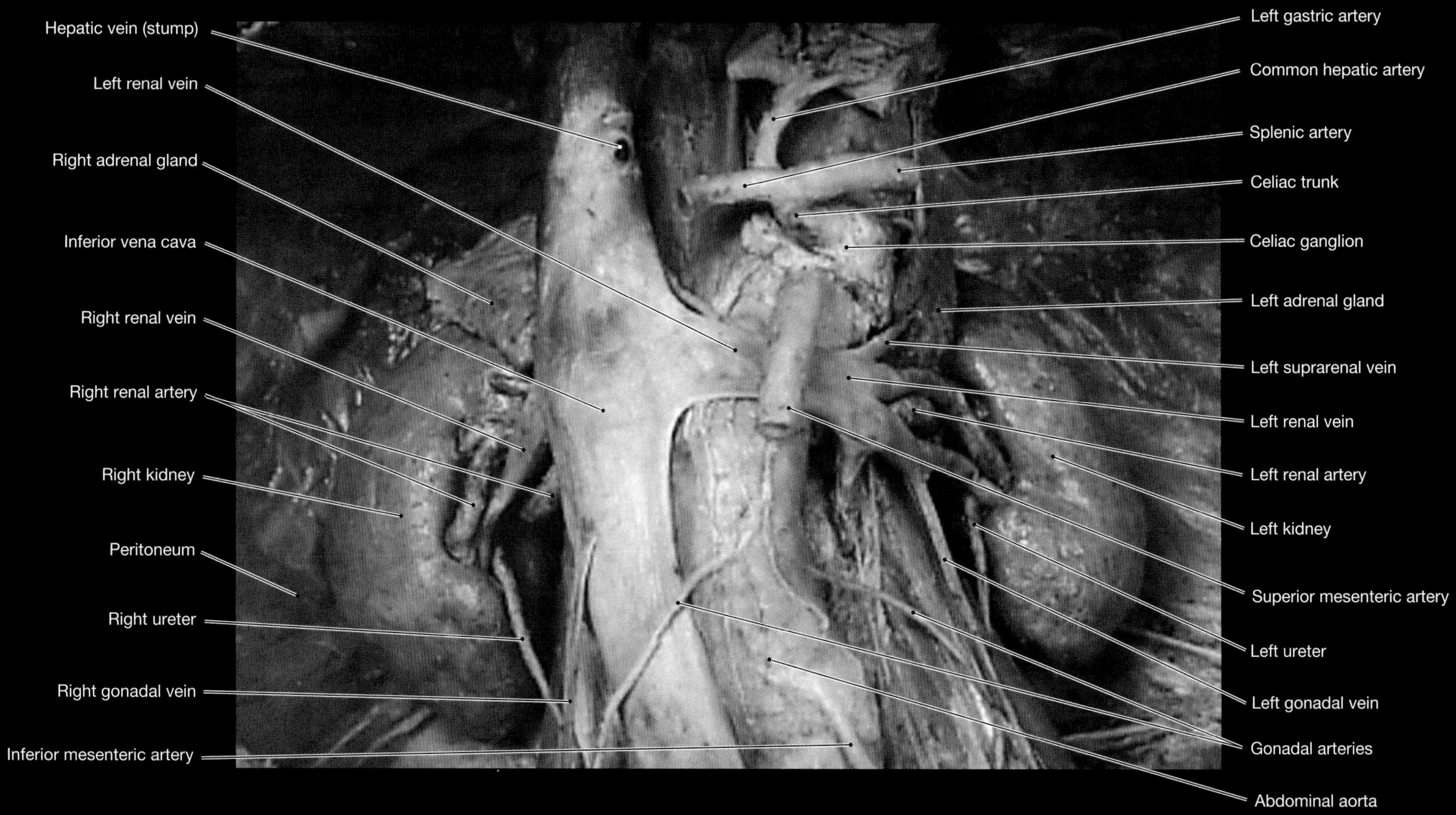

FIGURE 5.9   THE KIDNEYS AND ASSOCIATED STRUCTURES

Abdominal aorta

Gonadal arteries

Left gonadal vein

Left ureter

Superior mesenteric artery

Left kidney

Left renal artery

Left renal vein

Left suprarenal vein

Left adrenal gland

Celiac ganglion

Celiac trunk

Splenic artery

Common hepatic artery

Left gastric artery

Inferior mesenteric artery

Right gonadal vein

Right ureter

Peritoneum

Right kidney

Right renal artery

Right renal vein

Inferior vena cava

Right adrenal gland

Left renal vein

Hepatic vein (stump)

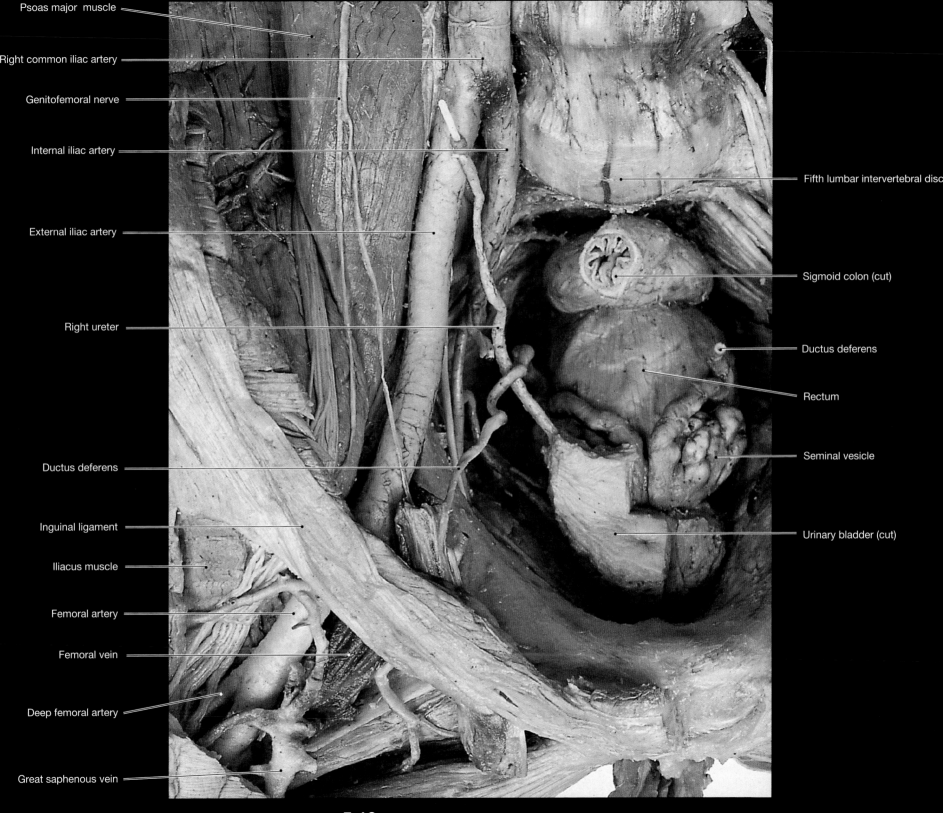

Psoas major muscle

Right common iliac artery

Genitofemoral nerve

Internal iliac artery

External iliac artery

Right ureter

Ductus deferens

Inguinal ligament

Iliacus muscle

Femoral artery

Femoral vein

Deep femoral artery

Great saphenous vein

Fifth lumbar intervertebral disc

Sigmoid colon (cut)

Ductus deferens

Rectum

Seminal vesicle

Urinary bladder (cut)

FIGURE **5.10a** THE INFERIOR PELVIS, SUPERIOR VIEW

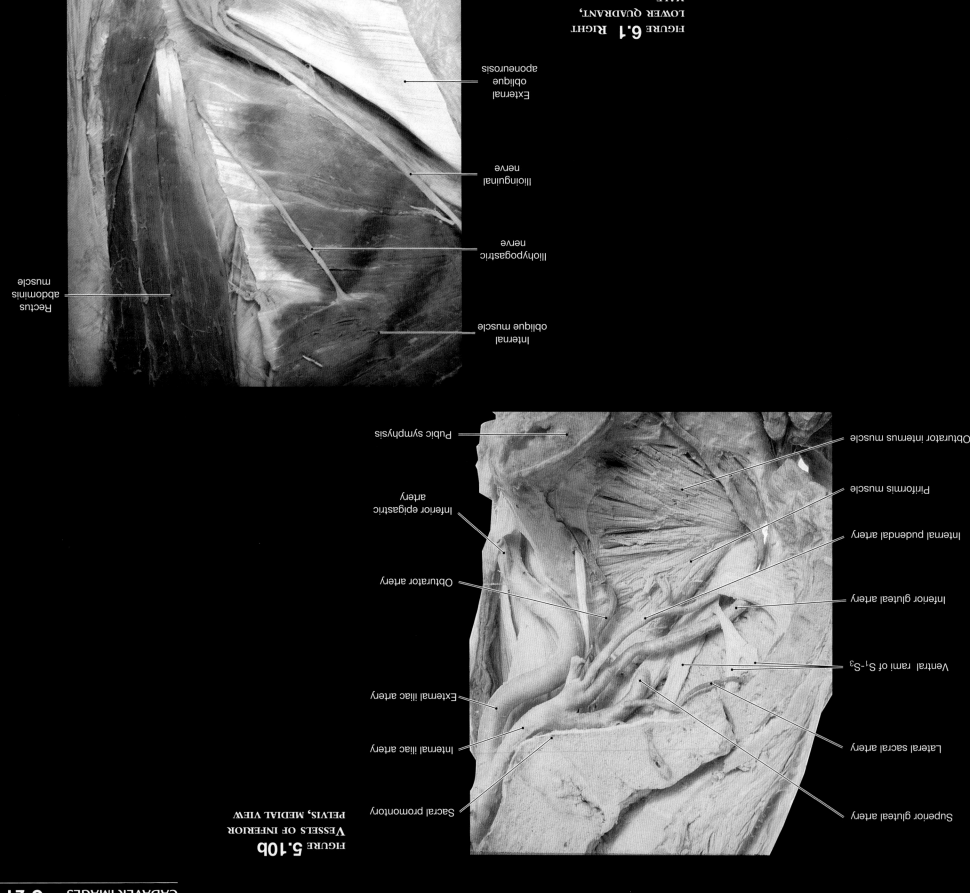

FIGURE 6.1 RIGHT
LOWER QUADRANT,
MALE

FIGURE 5.10b
VESSELS OF INFERIOR
PELVIS, MEDIAL VIEW

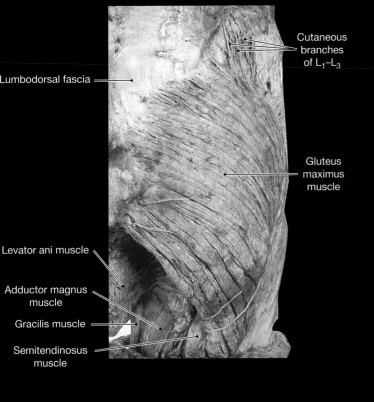

Cutaneous branches of L₁–L₃

Lumbodorsal fascia

Gluteus maximus muscle

Levator ani muscle

Adductor magnus muscle

Gracilis muscle

Semitendinosus muscle

FIGURE **6.2** RIGHT HIP, SUPERFICIAL DISSECTION, POSTERIOR VIEW

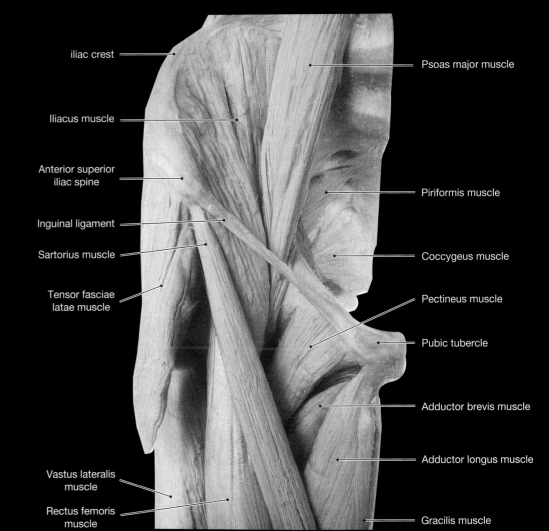

iliac crest

Iliacus muscle

Anterior superior iliac spine

Inguinal ligament

Sartorius muscle

Tensor fasciae latae muscle

Psoas major muscle

Piriformis muscle

Coccygeus muscle

Pectineus muscle

Pubic tubercle

Adductor brevis muscle

Adductor longus muscle

Vastus lateralis muscle

Rectus femoris muscle

Gracilis muscle

FIGURE **6.3** RIGHT HIP AND THIGH, ANTERIOR VIEW

FIGURE **6.4a** RIGHT
FOOT, SUPERFICIAL
DISSECTION, LATERAL
VIEW

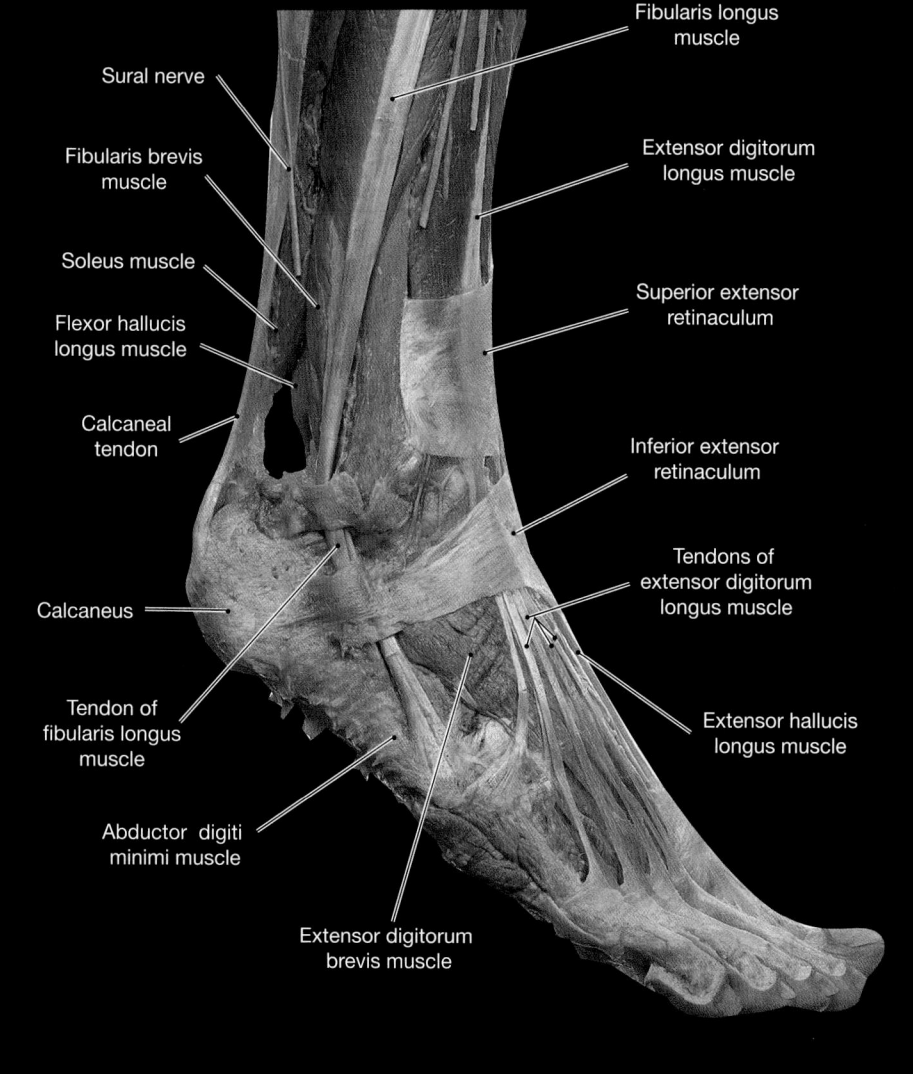

Sural nerve

Fibularis longus
muscle

Fibularis brevis
muscle

Extensor digitorum
longus muscle

Soleus muscle

Flexor hallucis
longus muscle

Superior extensor
retinaculum

Calcaneal
tendon

Inferior extensor
retinaculum

Calcaneus

Tendons of
extensor digitorum
longus muscle

Tendon of
fibularis longus
muscle

Extensor hallucis
longus muscle

Abductor digiti
minimi muscle

Extensor digitorum
brevis muscle

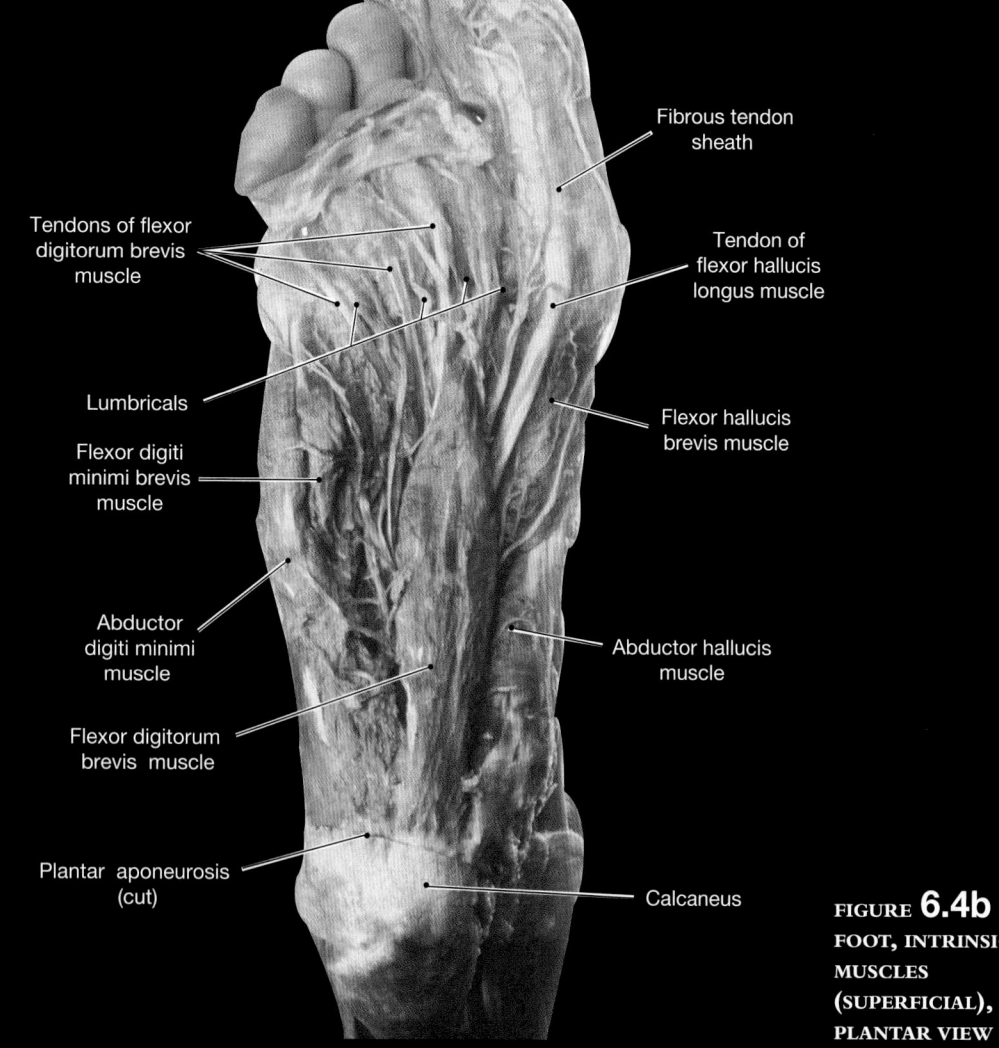

Fibrous tendon
sheath

Tendons of flexor
digitorum brevis
muscle

Tendon of
flexor hallucis
longus muscle

Lumbricals

Flexor digiti
minimi brevis
muscle

Flexor hallucis
brevis muscle

Abductor
digiti minimi
muscle

Abductor hallucis
muscle

Flexor digitorum
brevis muscle

Plantar aponeurosis
(cut)

Calcaneus

FIGURE **6.4b** RIGHT
FOOT, INTRINSIC
MUSCLES
(SUPERFICIAL),
PLANTAR VIEW

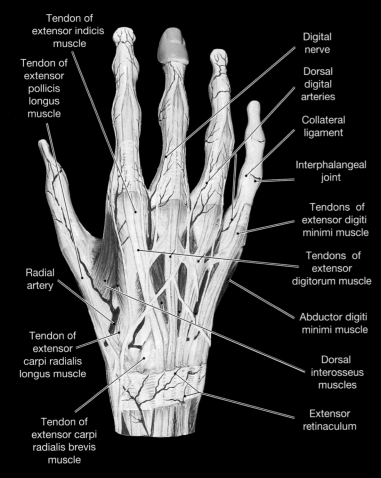

Tendon of extensor indicis muscle

Tendon of extensor pollicis longus muscle

Radial artery

Tendon of extensor carpi radialis longus muscle

Tendon of extensor carpi radialis brevis muscle

Digital nerve

Dorsal digital arteries

Collateral ligament

Interphalangeal joint

Tendons of extensor digiti minimi muscle

Tendons of extensor digitorum muscle

Abductor digiti minimi muscle

Dorsal interosseus muscles

Extensor retinaculum

FIGURE **6.5a** MODEL OF THE RIGHT HAND, POSTERIOR VIEW

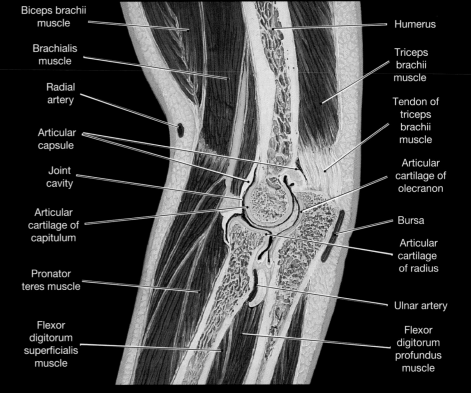

Biceps brachii muscle

Brachialis muscle

Radial artery

Articular capsule

Joint cavity

Articular cartilage of capitulum

Pronator teres muscle

Flexor digitorum superficialis muscle

Humerus

Triceps brachii muscle

Tendon of triceps brachii muscle

Articular cartilage of olecranon

Bursa

Articular cartilage of radius

Ulnar artery

Flexor digitorum profundus muscle

FIGURE **6.5b** MODEL OF THE ELBOW JOINT, LONGITUDINAL SECTION

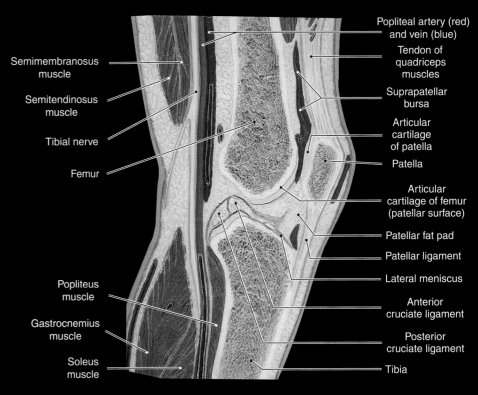

Semimembranosus muscle

Semitendinosus muscle

Tibial nerve

Femur

Popliteus muscle

Gastrocnemius muscle

Soleus muscle

Popliteal artery (red) and vein (blue)

Tendon of quadriceps muscles

Suprapatellar bursa

Articular cartilage of patella

Patella

Articular cartilage of femur (patellar surface)

Patellar fat pad

Patellar ligament

Lateral meniscus

Anterior cruciate ligament

Posterior cruciate ligament

Tibia

FIGURE **6.5c** MODEL OF THE KNEE JOINT, SAGITTAL SECTION

HISTOLOGY IMAGES

FIGURE 1.1   SIMPLE COLUMNAR EPITHELIUM WITH GOBLET CELLS (LM×480)   H-2

FIGURE 1.2   SIMPLE CUBOIDAL AND SIMPLE SQUAMOUS EPITHELIUM (LM×240)   H-2

FIGURE 1.3   STRATIFIED SQUAMOUS EPITHELIUM (LM×240) H-2

FIGURE 1.4   STRATIFIED COLUMNAR EPITHELIUM (LM×480) H-2

FIGURE 1.5   PSEUDOSTRATIFIED COLUMNAR EPITHELIUM (LM×480) H-2

FIGURE 1.6   TRANSITIONAL EPITHELIUM (URINARY BLADDER) (LM×480) . H-2

FIGURE 2.1   PANCREATIC ISLETS (ISLETS OF LANGERHANS) (LM×480) . . . H-3

FIGURE 2.2   AREOLAR CONNECTIVE TISSUE (MESENTERIC SPREAD)
(LM×480) H-3

FIGURE 2.3   DENSE IRREGULAR CONNECTIVE TISSUE (DERMIS OF THE SKIN)
(LM×480) H-3

FIGURE 2.4   TENDON (DENSE REGULAR CONNECTIVE TISSUE) (LM×240) . . H-3

FIGURE 2.5   HYALINE CARTILAGE (TRACHEA) (LM×240) H-3

FIGURE 2.6   ELASTIC CARTILAGE (AURICLE OF THE EAR) (ELASTIN STAIN)
(LM×480) H-3

FIGURE 3.1   FIBROCARTILAGE (PUBIC SYMPHYSIS) (LM×240) H-4

FIGURE 3.2   INTRAMEMBRANOUS (MEMBRANE) BONE DEVELOPMENT
(FETAL PIG) (LM×240) H-4

FIGURE 3.3   ENDOCHONDRAL OSSIFICATION AT THE EPIPHYSEAL CARTILAGE
(FETAL METATARSAL) (LM×48) H-4

FIGURE 3.4   BONE SPICULE WITHIN THE DIAPHYSIS OF DEVELOPING BONE
(LM×240) H-4

FIGURE 3.5   COMPACT BONE (CROSS SECTION), GROUND BONE (LM×120) . H-4

FIGURE 3.6   TRABECULAR (CANCELLOUS) BONE (LM×240) H-4

FIGURE 4.1   SKELETAL MUSCLE (CROSS SECTION) (LM×480) H-5

FIGURE 4.2   SKELETAL MUSCLE (LONGITUDINAL SECTION) (LM×480) H-5

FIGURE 4.3   CARDIAC MUSCLE (LM×480) H-5

FIGURE 4.4   SMOOTH MUSCLE (LONGITUDINAL AND CROSS SECTIONS)
(LM×480) H-5

FIGURE 4.5   CEREBELLUM (LM×120) H-5

FIGURE 4.6   PURKINJE CELLS OF THE CEREBELLUM (SILVER STAIN) (LM×480) . H-5

FIGURE 5.1   PERIPHERAL NERVE (CROSS SECTION) (LM×110) H-6

FIGURE 5.2   PURKINJE FIBERS WITHIN VENTRICLE OF HUMAN HEART
(LM×110) H-6

FIGURE 5.3   CROSS SECTION OF ARTERY AND VEIN (LM×110) H-6

FIGURE 5.4   CAPILLARIES WITHIN ADIPOSE TISSUE (LM×440) H-6

FIGURE 5.5   LUNG: TRANSITION FROM A TERMINAL BRONCHIOLE TO A
RESPIRATORY BRONCHIOLE (LM×65) H-6

FIGURE 5.6   LUNG: ALVEOLAR DUCT (LM×65) H-6

FIGURE 6.1   LUNG: PULMONARY ALVEOLI (LM×220) H-7

FIGURE 6.2   AGGREGATED LYMPHOID NODULES (PEYER'S PATCHES)
OF ILEUM (LM×120) H-7

FIGURE 6.3   LYMPH NODE (LM×120) H-7

FIGURE 6.4   THYMUS OF A CHILD WITH HASSALL'S CORPUSCLES (LM×120) H-7

FIGURE 6.5   ATROPHIC THYMUS OF AN ADULT (LM×120) H-7

FIGURE 6.6   SPLEEN (LM×120) H-7

FIGURE 7.1   KIDNEY CORTEX: RENAL CORPUSCLE, PROXIMAL AND DISTAL
CONVOLUTED TUBULES (LM×500) H-8

FIGURE 7.2   THYROID GLAND (LM×50) H-8

FIGURE 7.3   ENDOCRINE PANCREAS: PANCREATIC ISLETS (ISLETS OF
LANGERHANS) (LM×200) H-8

FIGURE 7.4   TESTIS (LM×50) H-8

FIGURE 7.5   PRIMORDIAL AND PRIMARY FOLLICLES WITHIN THE OVARY
(LM×50) H-8

FIGURE 7.6   GRAAFIAN FOLLICLE WITHIN THE OVARY (LM×50) H-8

FIGURE 8.1   FUNDUS OF STOMACH (LM×50) H-9

FIGURE 8.2   ILEUM OF SMALL INTESTINE (LM×50) H-9

FIGURE 8.3   COLON (LM×50) H-9

FIGURE 8.4   APPENDIX (LM×50) H-9

FIGURE 8.5   GALLBLADDER (LM×50) H-9

FIGURE 8.6   LIVER (LM×50) H-9

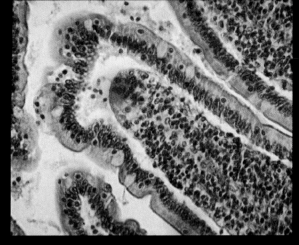

FIGURE **1.1** SIMPLE COLUMNAR EPITHELIUM WITH GOBLET CELLS (LM×480)

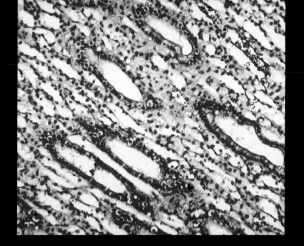

FIGURE **1.2** SIMPLE CUBOIDAL AND SIMPLE SQUAMOUS EPITHELIUM (LM×240)

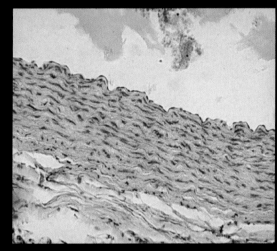

FIGURE **1.3** STRATIFIED SQUAMOUS EPITHELIUM (LM×240)

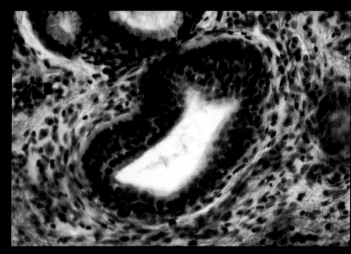

FIGURE **1.4** STRATIFIED COLUMNAR EPITHELIUM (LM×480)

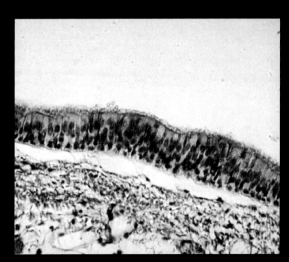

FIGURE **1.5** PSEUDOSTRATIFIED COLUMNAR EPITHELIUM (LM×480)

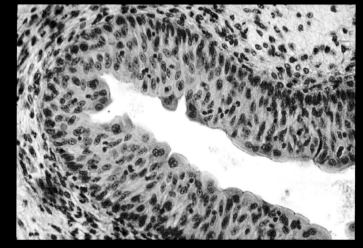

FIGURE **1.6** TRANSITIONAL EPITHELIUM (URINARY BLADDER) (LM×480)

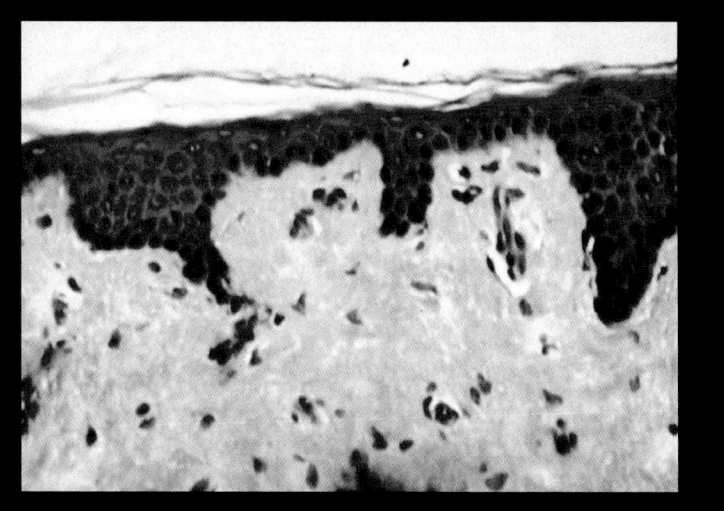

FIGURE **2.1** PANCREATIC ISLETS (ISLETS OF LANGERHANS) (LM×480)

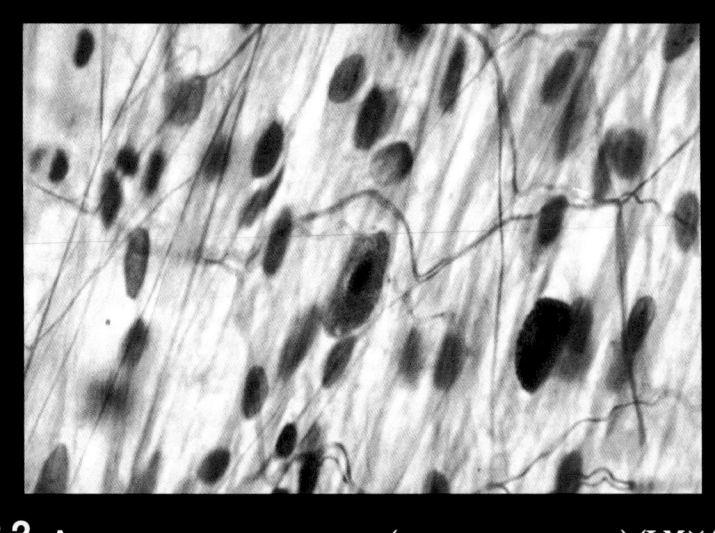

FIGURE **2.2** AREOLAR CONNECTIVE TISSUE (MESENTERIC SPREAD) (LM×480)

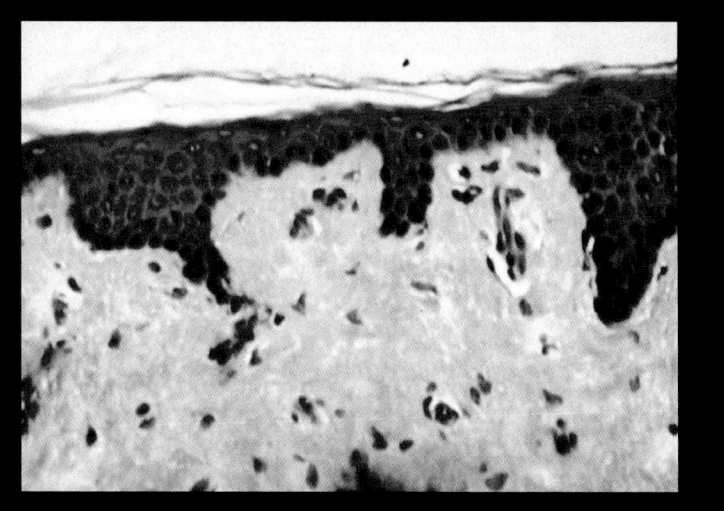

FIGURE **2.3** DENSE IRREGULAR CONNECTIVE TISSUE (DERMIS OF THE SKIN) (LM×480)

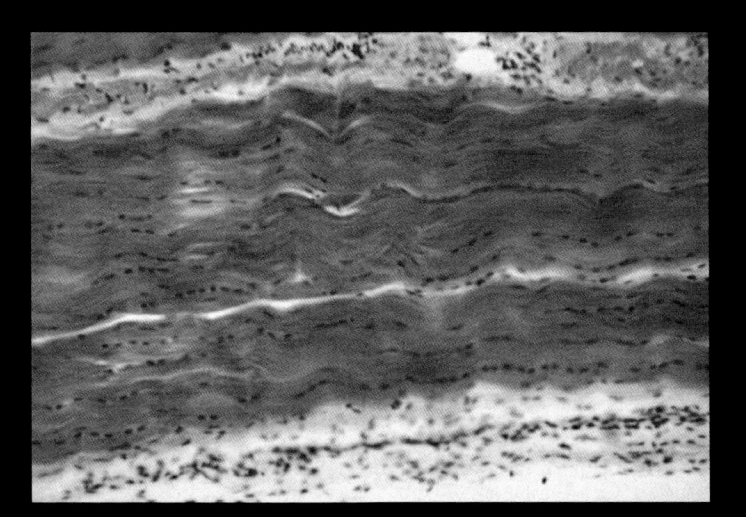

FIGURE **2.4** TENDON (DENSE REGULAR CONNECTIVE TISSUE) (LM×240)

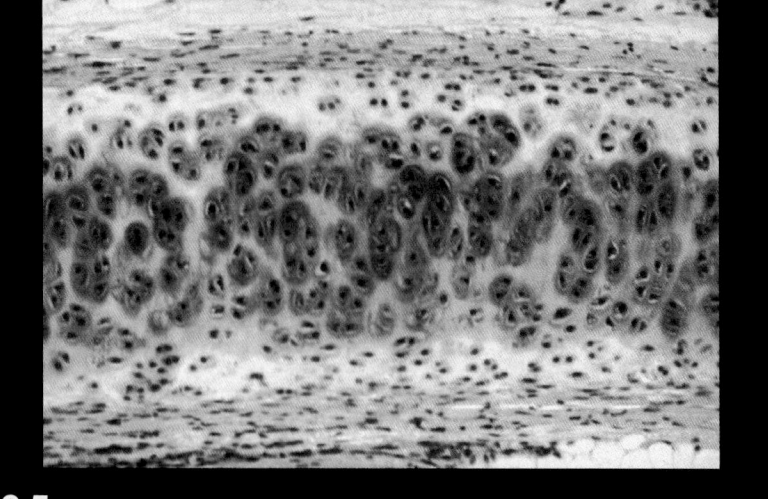

FIGURE **2.5** HYALINE CARTILAGE (TRACHEA) (LM×240)

FIGURE **2.6** ELASTIC CARTILAGE (AURICLE OF THE EAR) (ELASTIN STAIN) (LM×480)

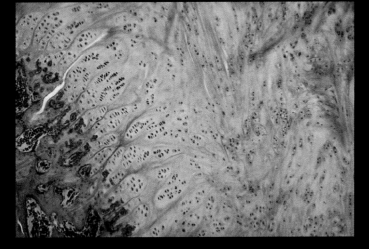

FIGURE **3.1** FIBROCARTILAGE (PUBIC SYMPHYSIS) (LM×240)

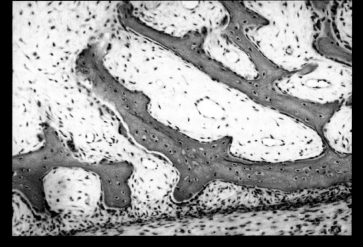

FIGURE **3.2** INTRAMEMBRANOUS (MEMBRANE) BONE DEVELOPMENT (FETAL PIG) (LM×240)

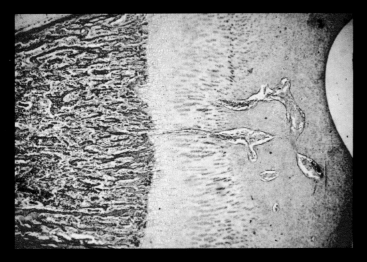

FIGURE **3.3** ENDOCHONDRAL OSSIFICATION AT THE EPIPHYSEAL CARTILAGE (FETAL METATARSAL) (LM×48)

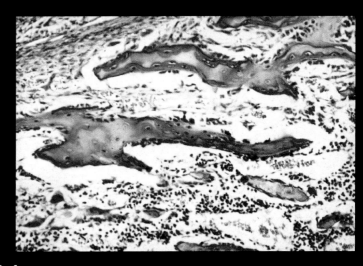

FIGURE **3.4** BONE SPICULE WITHIN THE DIAPHYSIS OF DEVELOPING BONE (LM×240)

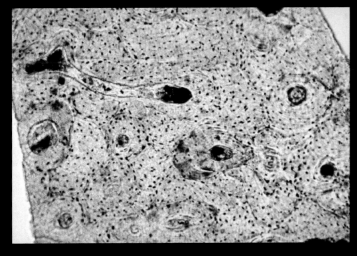

FIGURE **3.5** COMPACT BONE (CROSS SECTION), GROUND BONE (LM×120)

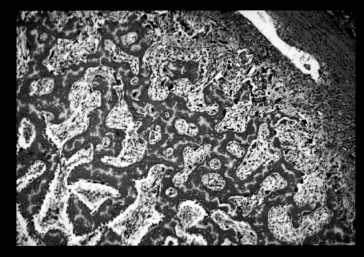

FIGURE **3.6** TRABECULAR (CANCELLOUS) BONE (LM×240)

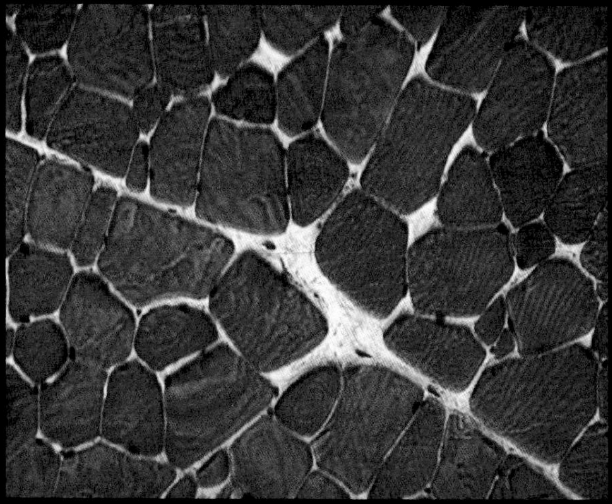

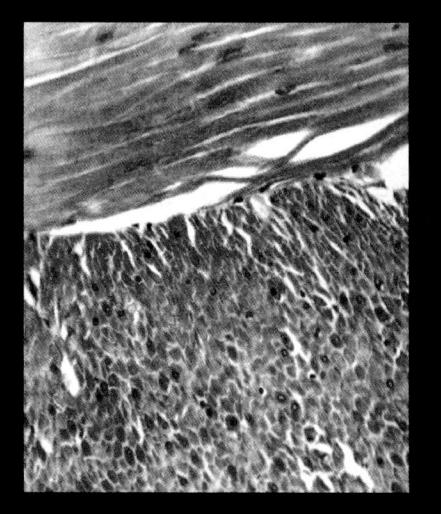

FIGURE **4.1** Skeletal muscle (cross section) (LM×480)

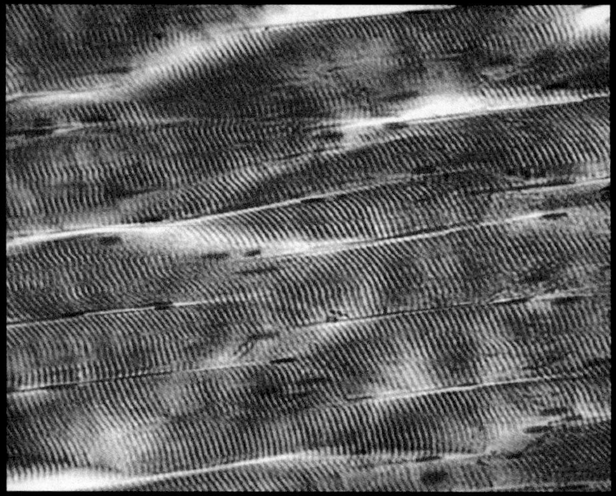

FIGURE **4.2** Skeletal muscle (longitudinal section) (LM×480)

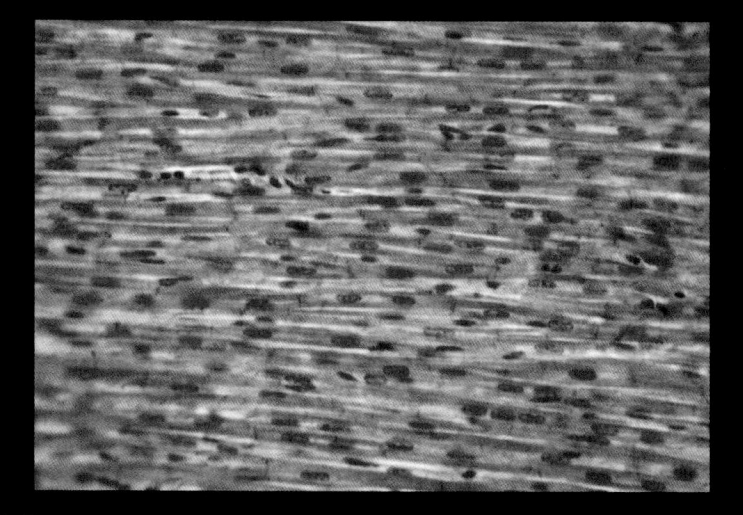

FIGURE **4.3** Cardiac muscle (LM×480)

FIGURE **4.4** Smooth muscle (longitudinal and cross sections) (LM×480)

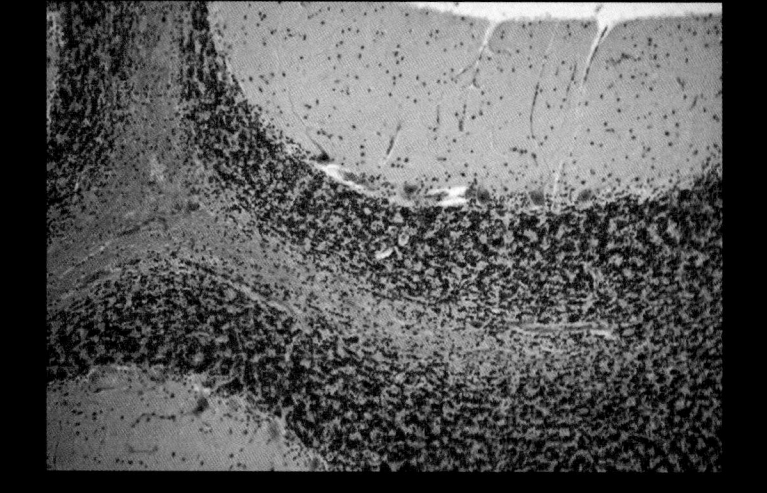

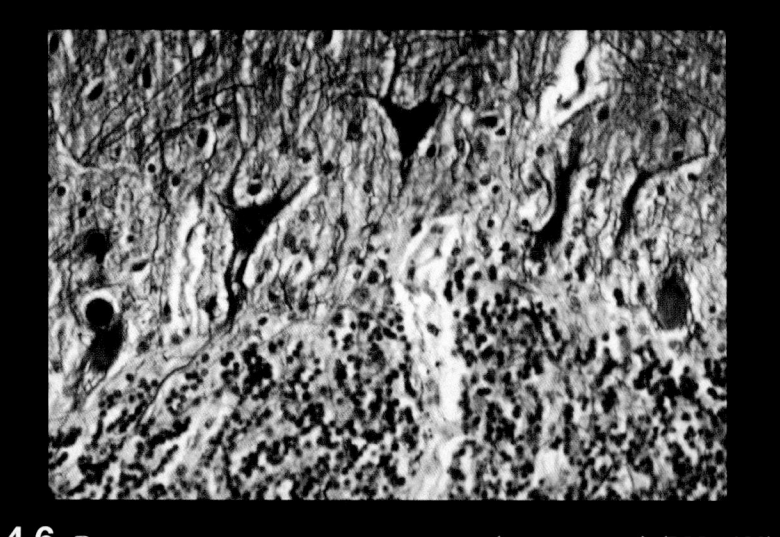

FIGURE **4.5** Cerebellum (LM×120)

FIGURE **4.6** Purkinje cells of the cerebellum (silver stain) (LM×480)

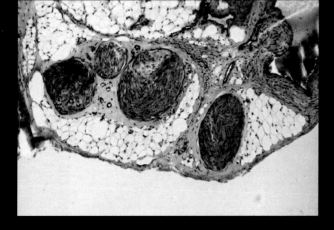

FIGURE **5.1** PERIPHERAL NERVE (CROSS SECTION) (LM×110)

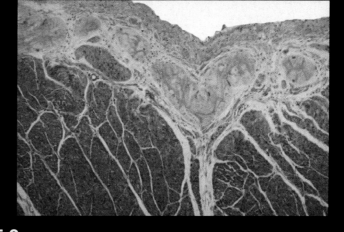

FIGURE **5.2** PURKINJE FIBERS WITHIN VENTRICLE OF HUMAN HEART (LM×110)

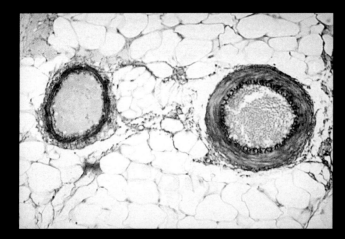

FIGURE **5.3** CROSS SECTION OF ARTERY AND VEIN (LM×110)

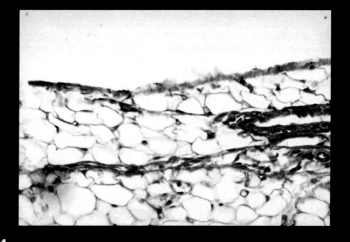

FIGURE **5.4** CAPILLARIES WITHIN ADIPOSE TISSUE (LM×440)

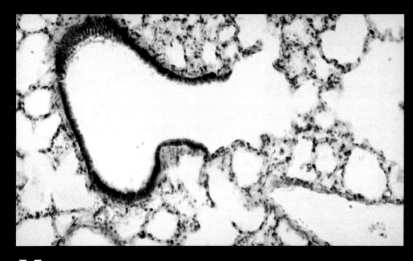

FIGURE **5.5** LUNG: TRANSITION FROM A TERMINAL BRONCHIOLE TO A RESPIRATORY BRONCHIOLE (LM×65)

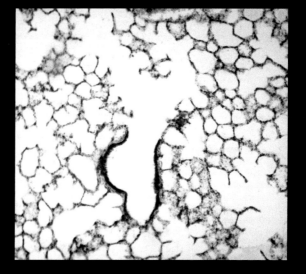

FIGURE **5.6** LUNG: ALVEOLAR DUCT (LM×65)

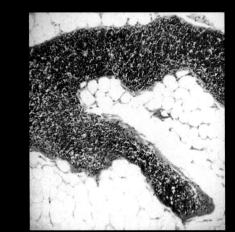

6.5 ATROPHIC THYMUS OF AN ADULT (LM×120)

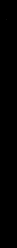

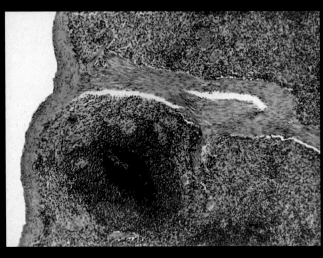

FIGURE 6.6 SPLEEN (LM×120)

6.3 LYMPH NODE (LM×120)

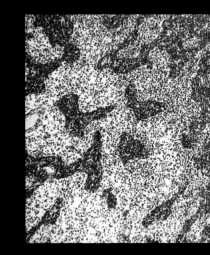

FIGURE 6.4 THYMUS OF A CHILD WITH HASSALL'S CORPUSCLES (LM×120)

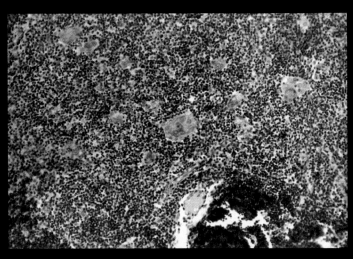

6.1 LUNG: PULMONARY ALVEOLI (LM×220)

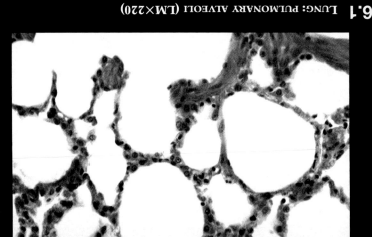

FIGURE 6.2 AGGREGATED LYMPHOID NODULES (PEYER'S PATCHES) OF ILEUM (LM×120)

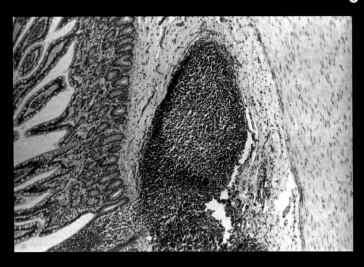

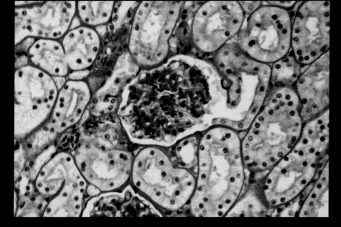

FIGURE **7.1** KIDNEY CORTEX: RENAL CORPUSCLE, PROXIMAL AND DISTAL CONVOLUTED TUBULES (LM×500)

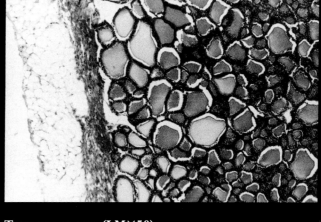

FIGURE **7.2** THYROID GLAND (LM×50)

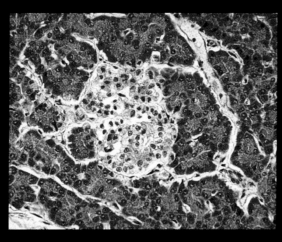

FIGURE **7.3** ENDOCRINE PANCREAS: PANCREATIC ISLETS (ISLETS OF LANGERHANS) (LM×200)

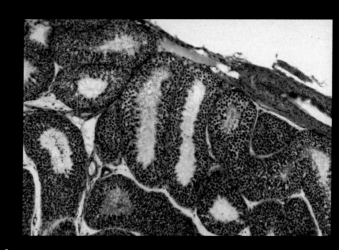

FIGURE **7.4** TESTIS (LM×50)

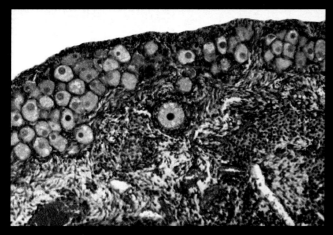

FIGURE **7.5** PRIMORDIAL AND PRIMARY FOLLICLES WITHIN THE OVARY (LM×50)

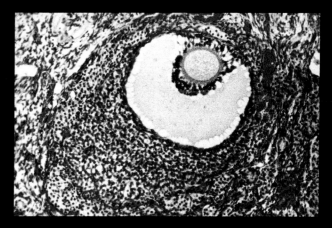

FIGURE **7.6** GRAAFIAN FOLLICLE WITHIN THE OVARY (LM×50)

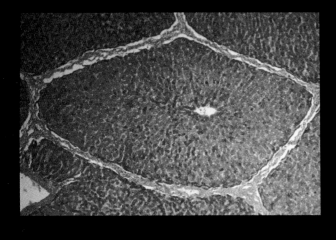

FIGURE 8.6 LIVER (LM×50)

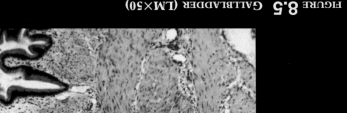

FIGURE 8.5 GALLBLADDER (LM×50)

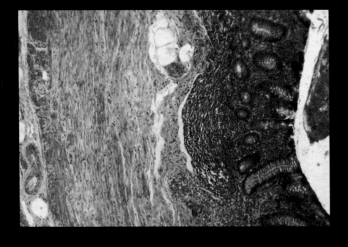

FIGURE 8.4 APPENDIX (LM×50)

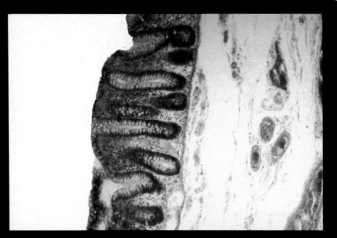

FIGURE 8.3 COLON (LM×50)

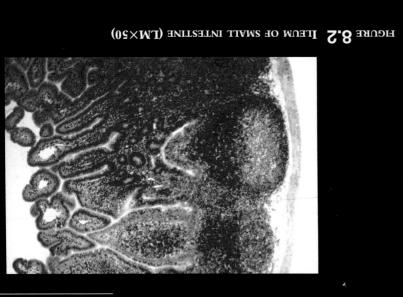

FIGURE 8.2 ILEUM OF SMALL INTESTINE (LM×50)

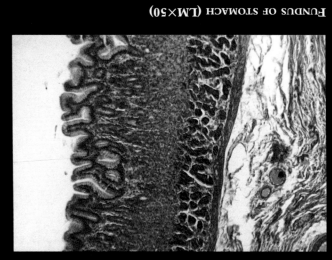

FIGURE 8.1 FUNDUS OF STOMACH (LM×50)